Eat, Drink, Heal:
The Art and Science of
Surgical Nutrition

Gregory A. Buford, MD FACS

Eat, Drink, Heal: The Art and Science of Surgical Nutrition

Printed by:
Core Aesthetics Publishing

Copyright © 2016, Gregory A. Buford, MD FACS

Published in the United States of America

Book ID: 160624-00451

ISBN-13: 978-1537132068
ISBN-10: 1537132067

This book is dedicated with love to my muses, Alicia, Ava, and Nikko.

Here's What's Inside...

Other books by Gregory A. Buford, MD FACS:

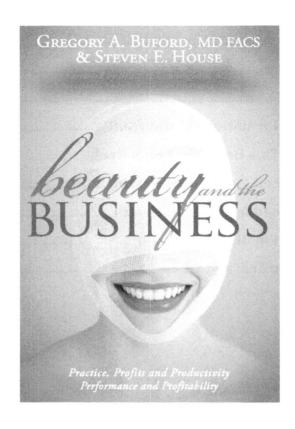

Testimonials

"Dr. Buford's book is an important tool for patients considering surgery. It is an exceptionally well-written and passionate argument to recognize the importance of nutrition in the perioperative period. Dr. Buford respects the intelligence of his readers and presents complex topics in an understandable way without overly simplifying the important points. I would recommend it to all of my patients considering surgery."

Alexander Z. Rivkin, MD
Facial Plastic Surgeon
Assistant Clinical Professor
David Geffen, UCLA School of Medicine

"The surgical experience is a journey that encompasses the preoperative preparation, the surgery day and surgical itself, and the recovery from two phases of healing; the acute phase of healing with swelling, bruising, and inflammation and the chronic or latent phase with repair, recovery, and remodeling. A mindful approach to surgery allows one the best chance of making this surgical experience or "journey" an enjoyable one. The keys to success are outlined in Dr. Buford's personal surgical 'recipe' book, **Eat, Drink and Heal…The Art of Surgical Nutrition***.*

Dr. Buford breaks down the micro and macronutrients that impact our daily health and can have a profound impact on surgical recovery and our general health. He goes further in what we also consider critical, in making the surgical experience one that goes beyond just conquering discomfort or swelling but is a chance to be in touch with one's body in the powerful triad of mind, soul, and body. Mindfulness during the surgical recovery offers patients a unique chance in a busy world to 'take a break', get in touch with what makes us who we are, and tap into the power that we have to impact our own health. This all starts with proper nutrition and exercise.

My advice: Follow Dr. Buford's 'living recipe' and experience your surgery by eating properly, positive thinking and finding inner strength, and finding peace...picking the right surgeon certainly helps also. "This handbook is helpful for anyone having surgery."

Corey S. Maas, MD, FACS
The Maas Clinic, San Francisco-Lake Tahoe
Associate Clinical Professor, University of CA, San Francisco

"Dr. Buford, a renowned plastic surgeon, addresses a subject which has largely gone ignored in western medicine. Educating patients in regard to nutrition is integral in both general health and post-operative healing. In our quick fix society dominated by reality television, the public is often misled into believing surgery is a fast way to improve health or appearance. In true reality, health starts with knowledge of a healthy diet and exercise. Dr. Buford provides an excellent foundation for explaining the important benefits of nutrition to optimize post-operative healing. He is comprehensive in his coverage of the subject, but masterfully simplifies the vast information to make it easy to understand. As a fellow surgeon, I believe he has bridged an important gap to empower patients and allow them to achieve their best health and surgical results. I feel this is a must read for patients and surgeons alike."

John P. Fezza, MD
Oculoplastic Surgeon, Sarasota, Florida

"Finally, a surgeon brings us more up to date on how to eat and supplement properly for surgery. Dr. Buford presents the information in a way that is accessible and practical."

Ben Gonzalez, MD
Founder and Medical Director
Atlantis Medical Wellness Center

"It's surprising that so few patients and physicians consider the major role nutrition plays in our overall health and well-being. In times of severe stress for our bodies, such as recovering from surgery, the importance of proper nutrition is even greater. In this book, Dr. Buford has given us a comprehensive and helpful guide for a better and healthier recovery. Patients and surgeons alike should read this book."

Jeffrey A. Raval, MD, MBA
Facial Plastic Surgeon Denver, Colorado

"Food is the fuel on which the human body runs. The quality of diet affects every aspect of health, from how well we heal and recover after surgery to how well we feel, and look, every day. By addressing the link between nutrition and outcomes in cosmetic surgery, Greg Buford is addressing an essential but neglected topic in medicine, and providing an important contribution."

David L. Katz, MD, MPH, FACPM, FACP, FACLM
Director, Yale University Prevention Research Center
Clinical Instructor, Yale University School of Medicine
President, American College of Lifestyle Medicine
Founder, True Health Initiative

"The importance of nutrition in surgery is just beginning to be recognized, not just by patients, but by their doctors. Dr. Buford has firmly established himself as a leader in this field. If you want to maximize your surgical results and heal as quickly as possible, Dr. Buford has compiled a must-read book!"

Brian Eichenberg, MD
Plastic Surgeon - Murrieta, California

"Dr. Buford does an excellent job in detailing the information that is lacking in our medical school education about the newest concepts in nutrition. Not only does healing after surgery depend on a person's physical well-being and nutritional status, it also depends on their overall ability to do self-care which includes appropriate nutrition, life balancing, and poor habit minimization. His matter-of-fact approach to these concepts educates the patient and the physician, which will likely enhance further the physician-patient relationship."

Nancy Thurman-Watson, MD, CPC, ELI-MP
Anesthesiologist, Certified Professional Career Coach

"I would like to commend Greg Buford, M.D. for taking the time to write this monograph on surgical nutrition. This is a magnificent book that covers the particulars of orally-based surgical nutrition in order to enhance recovery and well-being.

While most plastic surgeons operate on relatively healthy individuals, there are individuals who seek both aesthetic and reconstructive plastic surgery who have metabolic issues that increase risk of adverse events and a prolonged recovery. Requisite pre-surgery metabolic testing and nutritional support of deficiencies is good advice by Dr. Buford.

Like Dr. Buford, I agree that nutritional support of the surgical patient gets very little attention by most physicians who are not involved with burns, trauma, or major gastrointestinal surgery. Conversely, patients are also poorly educated with regards to diet, hydration, and foods that prove difficult to digest in the perioperative period.

In my own experience, recovery can be enhanced with simple steps that are outlined in this book regarding hydration, macronutrients, micronutrients, and probiotics. Patients appreciate nutritional advice that's practical and can be continued after recovery that will help enhance wellness.

Nutrition in everyday life also receives little attention, given the unhealthy eating habits of most Americans. Many individuals have little insight into the negative effect of what they eat on their health and wellness, not to mention maintenance of normal weight. This book gives great guidance to avoid fad diets, erroneous assumptions about foods, and ways to obtain additional education on nutrition. **Eat, Drink and Heal...The Art of Surgical Nutrition** *is a must read. It is both thought-provoking and solution-oriented."*

Mark L. Jewell, MD
Eugene, Oregon
Past President, The American Society for Aesthetic Plastic Surgery
Associate Clinical Professor, Plastic Surgery, Oregon Health Science University

Foreword

Healing after surgery may be the most important aspect of the entire operation, which starts with the initial presentation of the condition and ends with a long-term successful outcome and a friend being referred for another procedure. The entire process lasts months, if not a year or more. There are many critical steps in the process on the day of surgery, and much happens during a short period. However, the myriad of less obvious components are equally essential to excellence in surgery. None are more important than the comprehensive approach to diet, nutrition, and healing from within. And none are more representatively under-appreciated and taught.

Paying attention to a subject not emphasized adequately, Dr. Gregory A. Buford, MD, FACS has advanced our preparation and set the tone for improved outcomes in his book, with contributions by John Friedstein, CN (nutritionist). Healing from within can be the difference between a bad result and a good result, or even life and death from a serious injury like extensive, third-degree burns.

What is less apparent is how it can also be the difference between a good result and an excellent result in an aesthetic procedure. Aesthetic procedures and surgeries have surged in popularity in the last several decades. Essentially, they have become part of "lifestyle choices" and less considered "medical procedures". With this success, they have become commonplace, part of the popular culture, less risky and more casual. Diet, nutrition, and exercise have become a part of this story but are still somewhat neglected. While everyone knows something about the topic, many are confused about conflicting information and can't put the pieces together into a coherent program.

Dr. Buford walks us through the various stages of surgery, from start to finish. He explains the importance and role of macronutrients and basic food groups, as well as how they must be balanced.

Then he pieces together the importance of various micronutrients, vitamins, supplements, herbals, fruits, and vegetables. He produces a guideline for "race day" in his racecar analogy and discusses formulas for success. Then he guides us through the steps for healing and recovering from surgery. There is enough detail for some, but not enough to overwhelm those who just desire safe and useful guidelines. He explains how a change in medicine is continuing and how nutrition is a part of the story. Finally, he provides a wealth of resources for further study.

If nothing else, eat a balanced diet, and use the pages starting with micronutrients and supplements around the time of your procedure. Share this with your doctor, friends, and family. The information is invaluable and will undoubtedly improve the way you feel and heal. This book serves as a quick, useful handbook or travel guide for your procedure. Don't leave home without it!!

Brian M. Kinney, MD, FACS, MSME
Clinical Associate Professor of Plastic Surgery
University of Southern California (USC)
Parliamentarian, International Society of Plastic Regenerative Surgery (ISPRES)

As a world-renowned sports nutrition expert and nutrition researcher, Fortune 100 Corporations count on me to navigate them through the complex, confusing and at times downright confounding space of nutrition.

And as an expert performance coach, my world class pro-athletes rely on me to ensure they are in peak performance mode. One of the most important aspects of performance begins with recovery. Recovery nutrition is preparatory nutrition. My athletes will attest to the emphasis I place on ensuring they have the necessary, vital nutrients to speed optimal recovery and prepare them for the next challenge, mental or physical.

Whether you are a world-class athlete putting your career on the line, or a busy mom preparing for life enhancing surgery, recovery is job one. And job one for optimal recovery is nourishing your body with the healthy, nutrient rich foods and supplements that make the demanding work of healing easy for your body.

In the book, Eat, Drink & Heal, Dr. Buford presents an intelligent, scientifically supported and—dare I say—long overdue case for the role of nutrition in the healing process. As he says, while doctors must own their responsibility for the procedure, patients seeking the best possible outcome must also be accountable.

That means fueling your body with an abundance of the vital nutrients to promote health and wellbeing before your surgery and speed healing and recovery after.

What most excites me about this book from Dr. Buford is that it is here—it exists, finally. My work and my life revolve around the optimal application of nutrition and key nutritional supplements to support your best life. The information presented here, in this book, is solid, sound and accepted truth.

Yet, it is not lost on me that in the world of general medicine and cosmetic surgery these vital truths are for the most part completely ignored or overlooked.

I celebrate the continued integration of medicine—the growing and essential move to a more holistic approach to wellness and recovery. And I suspect that as most every pioneer does, Dr. Buford will face resistance, perhaps even attacks from an old guard of medicine which does not understand and/or is not willing to accept the the essential nature of healing nutrition.

No question the resistance to this knowledge will pass as the information becomes more widely known and understood. Your responsibility, as a patient, is your own best outcome. The good news is that here in your hands you hold a very comprehensive and yet simple-to-apply guide to the foods, fluid and even supplements which have been scientifically supported to help your body heal better, stronger, faster.

Oh yes, and after your doctor shares his/her shock at the speed and strength of your recovery, please feel free to share this book with them. For this is the best, fastest way to spread this quality information: from one doctor to the many patients.

To Your Health, Happiness and Healing~

Douglas Kalman, PhD, RD
Sports Nutritionist - Florida International University
Nutrition research Director, QPS (Miami Research Associates)
Co-Founder International Society of Sports Nutrition

12

Preface

Writing a book is a labor of love and often a process that takes on a mind of its own as words flow onto paper. This book was written not only to provide information, but also to affect a change in how we treat patients before and after surgery, and also in how patients treat themselves. The simple act of healing is far more than simple and requires a myriad of ingredients to accomplish a positive outcome. I set out not only to provide information to both doctors and patients, but also to challenge an institution that can be slow to change and a group of individuals who may not have the time or the resources to gather this information on their own.

The motivation for this book came from many sources, but I would be remiss if I failed to give credit to a few select people who truly inspired me to share the power of proper nutrition. My parents raised me to appreciate healthy, clean food. I will be forever grateful for their role in laying down a mindset that appreciates not only the joy of a properly made meal, but also the power of the ingredients that go into making it. I learned the basics of cooking as a young child and built upon this foundation as I grew older, but I never forgot the amazing meals that I consumed as a child and still do when I return home.

Now that I have grown a bit older, I look forward to passing along this same wisdom to my family. I owe a huge debt of gratitude to my fiancé, Alicia, for not only inspiring me to cook and cook often but also for consuming meals when they didn't always turn out as perfect as expected. And I need to thank her kids, Ava and Nikko, for their part in helping me shop and prepare the basics for these meals, as well as their constant curiosity about different fruits, vegetables, and so forth, which has led to many a very interesting combination on our dinner plates.

Finally, a big thanks goes out to my buddy Jorgen, who is never without the right bottle of delicious wine to go with that perfect grilled steak and veggies.

We've cracked a few bottles in our day, and I look forward to many more. A good friend who will cook with you is rare and a blessing. Hold on to those friends!

To the many other people who have inspired me, from professional chefs on Food Network to chefs in our local restaurants, who simply took the time to chat with me about what they do, I thank you. You are all artists and truly an inspiration!

I hope you enjoy reading this book as much as I enjoyed writing it. Bon appétit!

Greg

Why This Information Is Important

"Let food be thy medicine and medicine be thy food."
- **Hippocrates** (philosopher)

The Problem and Why You Should Care

Imagine a racetrack. Cars are ready to enter. Before they do, they are checked from head to toe—engines scrutinized for the smallest defect or deficiency, and all factors considered for the drive ahead. No driver would ever enter his car without this check, knowing that any missed item, any single problem, no matter how small, could mean the difference between not only winning and losing but also his exiting the car in one piece.

Now, imagine your operation. Every move of your surgeon's hand is calculated and precise, every action intentional. You lie supine on the operating table, your body awaiting the first incision. When the surgery is over, you are taken to the recovery room, where the real journey begins—the journey of healing. What will set the stage for success or for failure has, in many ways, already been decided as a result of actions taken or not taken before you even entered the operating room.

You were prepared. Knowing that after surgery your body would be sent into metabolic overdrive, you prepared by eating healthy, balanced meals in the weeks before and supplemented with essential micronutrients necessary for optimal healing. You knew what was necessary. You prepared and were ready for what lay ahead.

As the weeks pass after surgery, your energy levels rapidly improve, your incisions heal without problems, and you eventually return to your normal life. Your decision to proactively prepare made all the difference in the world, but you are an exception; this is not what normally happens. Your doctor prepared for this surgery for a good part of his life. His training provided him the latest and greatest in technology and the means to get you safely in and out of surgery. What he was not prepared for is one of the most critical elements to healing itself and something that much of the medical profession refuses to acknowledge as critical to the process of healing.

The medical profession is so focused on technology that it has left behind, and seemingly ignored, one of the most basic elements that can determine the course and the quality of your healing.

In the training curriculum of the top ten medical schools today (as ranked by U.S. News and World Report), only six allotted time to courses that included some focus on nutrition. While there was some emphasis, this information was supplied more in the form of "Curriculum Threads", as opposed to a formal course dedicated to this critical topic. Despite the proven impact of a healthy diet on our bodies under normal conditions, the American medical profession treats its patients with nutritional standards that are outdated, washed-up, and grossly out of sync with the ever-growing database of knowledge regarding nutrition. This outdated information is being taught to our young physicians.

The question that must be asked: Why? Why do we continue to ignore data and devalue the importance of proper nutrition as a means for optimal healing?

There are several reasons, but one of the most apparent is the fact that with an ever-expanding base of knowledge, medical schools must focus on what they deem to be the most essential and filter out that which they regard as less important. Therein lies the problem. Medical school administrators simply do not see nutrition as critical to the training of physicians, and so these young minds are left to gather and assimilate this information on their own once released into private practice.

The interesting twist to this is that more and more physicians are stepping away from convention and taking the lead on their own in guiding their patients to improved outcomes and smoother recoveries by incorporating programs before and after surgery to promote healing. These doctors are the exception and not the rule.

The sad fact is that several factors block more global adoption of this strategy, and threaten to do so for years to come, and to do so in combination with other factors which make it even more critical that patients are well-nourished both before and after their procedures.

The first problem is the global lack of emphasis on the importance of surgical nutrition. Little time, if any, is spent on educating the medical student on nutrition, and even less is spent once these young doctors are actively practicing medicine. Most doctors are simply too busy to spend time both educating their patients and educating themselves on what really works and what doesn't, so the same tired information is passed on from generation to generation.

Not only do we not know what we don't know about nutrition, but we also don't have the financial motivation to change our ways. There is little to no reimbursement for teaching our patients about proper nutrition. In addition, because there is no financial motivation for big drug companies to research supplements, this area is a big unknown and will no doubt remain so for years to come. There is data that shows efficacy but it is sparse, often questioned, and seen as suspect by the allopathic branch of the medical profession. As physicians continue to see more patients and get paid less, the pure and simple fact is that nutrition will never be a priority.

As costs associated with healthcare continue to rise, more surgeries are being performed on an outpatient basis in an effort to improve both cost and time-efficiency. With this rapid discharge, a greater burden is placed on both the patient and their immediate caregiver with respect to management of nutritional intake during this critical period of healing. This issue alone has the potential to increase the risk for early complications and compromise optimal outcomes.

In addition, during the early post-operative period, surgical patients are in pain and often have very little appetite.

They are usually on a number of medications, which makes it challenging for them to prepare healthy meals and potentially reduces their interest in solid food. In addition, given the vast amount of information related to nutrition online and through the media, a majority of patients are often confused and literally paralyzed when it comes to making healthy choices. The result? Many eat poorly; some eat little to nothing at all. In so doing, their bodies are robbed of important building blocks for the repairs that are essential for healing during this critical period.

Add to this the fact that before surgery, we doctors typically provide you with little to no nutritional guidance. As previously mentioned, we are not only poorly trained in the area of surgical nutrition, but, quite simply, we do not have the time, the interest, or the appreciation for the importance of early postoperative nutrition. Even the best surgical training programs continue to place little value on nutrition, and instead, choose to focus on technical aspects of surgery and the growing importance of cost-containment.

When issues do arise, they often present in the form of wound-healing complications and sub-optimal results. These complications not only increase healing time but may also compromise the quality of life. The end result is that a surgical procedure performed by a talented surgeon on a motivated patient may ultimately lead to a sub-optimal result, simply because the proper nutrients were not available during the early phases of healing.

To optimally heal, proper building blocks need to be made available, not only after surgery but also before surgery so that each patient is adequately prepared for the procedure itself. This requires education, planning, and the recognition of the importance of surgical nutrition.

The medical system needs to change from the ground up, not only with regard to educating our doctors, but also with regard to the education of our patients. We need to improve how we approach surgery from the standpoint of the surgeon as well as the patient, and both sides ultimately need to bear responsibility for outcomes. It is no longer acceptable to simply play naive and cross our fingers. The time has come for a paradigm shift, and we must move forward in a manner that is both responsible and reasonable and that benefits both parties.

This book is a wake-up call to your doctor as well as to you, the consumer. What you do with it can make all the difference to your health.

Why I Am So Passionate About Nutrition

As a plastic surgeon, I was trained to see patients, assess their needs, offer them the latest and greatest in products and procedures, and then whisk them on their merry way to new-and-improved appearances. Only recently did it dawn on me that there is far more to success in healing than the latest technology and that the key to optimal results may actually reside within my patients themselves and not on something external.

Growing up in Oregon, I was raised to appreciate the value of good nutrition and healthy food. My parents rarely, if ever, purchased anything in a box and made most of our meals from scratch, beginning with high-quality ingredients.

While I strayed from this level of quality during my college and medical school years, I eventually returned to a healthier pattern of eating after I realized just what I had done to my body by ingesting the average American diet. In my early 40s, I found myself out of shape, out of energy, working too hard, and feeling less well than I had in years. At this point, I realized that I needed to make a change. If I continued down this path, like most middle-aged men, I would be on the typical slew of medications, heading toward an early death with compromised quality of life in the years in between.

I didn't like this option. And so I changed.

I changed the way I ate, I hired a personal trainer, and I ultimately went on to compete in a local Men's Physique Competition, where I took first place in the Men's Masters (over 45) category in addition to a fifth-place finish in the Overall and Novice Class.

What I learned was the transformative power of focused exercise and, far more importantly, the impact of a good, clean diet. I found that results were based far more on what I ate than on what I did at the gym.

I incorporated this knowledge into the management of my body contouring patients. I began testing their nutritional fitness before surgery and found that many of them had deficiencies that, if left untreated, could potentially hamper their ability to achieve optimal healing. I also found that by incorporating the patient into their own care, they were more vested and more likely to be compliant, both before and after surgery, with respect to their nutritional needs. Patients were eager to participate in this type of process if it meant that they might be able to not only improve their immediate outcomes but also maintain these results over time.

Then one day my fiancé was diagnosed with thyroid cancer. Although the process was familiar to me, having completed a general surgery residency and having actually performed a number of thyroid surgeries in the past, what was not evident to me was how woefully inadequate we are at teaching our patients what and how to eat following surgery. Let me state clearly that her surgeon was amazingly gifted and undoubtedly saved her life, but where he excelled in surgical prowess, he and his staff could have gone further in instructing patients on what and how they should eat to potentiate their ability to heal properly. To his credit, that is a fault that we as surgeons are all guilty of. Given the direction in which the American healthcare system is heading, it is a fault that will no doubt be replicated and passed down for generations of surgeons to come.

That is why I am writing this book and why I am so passionate about optimal nutrition for surgical patients. The road to optimal wellness is often challenging and requires dedication, but when the endpoint is a more productive and vigorous life, and when the years ahead are potentially free of disease, there is no greater reward.

In purchasing this book and in completing the introduction, you have taken the first step to a healthier and more fulfilling life. I challenge you to use this resource as a roadmap to identify areas in which you feel strong and areas in which you do not. Life is an amazing thing and must be cherished. If we truly only go around one time, then that time must matter and no opportunity go unused.

How to Use This Book Most Effectively

This book is designed to be a guide for you not only before your surgery, but also for the rest of your life. How you eat determines both how you heal and the course of your overall health. To better understand how to effectively use this information, let's talk about its organization and what you really need to focus on.

The book is structured into the following segments:

- **Why This Information Is Important**
- **What You Need for Optimal Healing**
- **What You Need for Optimal Health**
- **How You Can Learn More About Proper Nutrition**

The first section (**Why This Information Is Important**) lays the groundwork and explains not only how and why proper nutrition is important for healing, but also expresses the underlying reasons for writing this book. Start here so that you understand the basic premise behind the book itself, as well as the ultimate direction of its contents.

The following section (**What You Need for Optimal Healing**) is critical for anyone undergoing surgery anytime soon. You need to read this information and digest it (no pun intended) accordingly. This is the stuff that will help you heal better and help make your recovery as smooth as possible. Read this information carefully and thoughtfully, and take good notes. Use it to prepare for your surgery, and definitely share it with your surgeon.

The next section (**What You Need for Optimal Health**) provides a foundation for attaining and maintaining long-term health.
While this chapter is informative, you can read it after the prior essential chapter related to surgical healing, but definitely read it at some point. It's essential!

The concluding section (**How You Can Learn More**) provides a broad array of information that will help you stay current in the various aspects of optimal nutrition and serves as a reference point. This can be read last.

Like most of you, I have started reading many books, only to become overwhelmed and ultimately put them down after the initial few chapters. I don't want you to do this. Please feel free to skip forward to essential chapters and return to any peripheral information at a later time. But use this information. If you do, it can have very positive effects on the course of your surgery and the healing period that follows.

A wise man once said, "In the end, it's not the years in your life that count; it's the life in your years." Although I am hopefully nowhere near the end, I would have to agree with him completely. Be well, and enjoy the rest of the book. It just may change your life...if you let it!

What You Need for Optimal Healing

"God, in His infinite wisdom, neglected nothing and if we would eat our food without trying to improve, change or refine it, thereby destroying its life-giving elements; it would meet all requirements of the body."
 - **Jethro Kloss** (holistic healer)

The Importance of Supplements:

Leaving your post-operative course to chance isn't the best option. You need to prepare for the time after surgery long before the surgery itself, and how well you plan could mean the difference between a speedy recovery and one that is fraught with complications.

While there are a number of supplements that you can take both before and after your surgery, you will most likely be taking a number of medications, so the goal is to keep your list as simple as possible. I would suggest the following regimen as a starting point. From here, you are welcome to add additional supplements as you see fit, and as your doctor recommends. As noted in the previous chapters, some supplements (while beneficial for your health) may have effects (such as blood thinning), which will require you to either limit or avoid them altogether, depending upon your overall health, as well as the procedure that you plan to undergo. I recommend the following plan for optimal healing.

Take at least two weeks before surgery:

- Multi-vitamin (Take as directed)
- Vitamin D3 (1,000 to 2,000 IU/day)
- Vitamin K2 (180-200 mcg/day)
- L-Thiamine (100 mg: 1 in the afternoon and 1 before sleep)
- Relora (250 mg: 1 tablet three times/day)
- CoQ-10 – Ubiquinol form (200 mg: 1 tablet/day)
- Methylated B-12 (1,000 mg: 1 tablet/day)
- Quercetin (500-2,000 mg/day)
- L-Glutamine (5-10 g/day)
- L-Citrulline (2-6 g/day)
- Boswellia Serrata (150-250 mg tablets: 2-3 times per day)

- Probiotic (Look for a supplement containing at least five strains of beneficial bacteria)
- Cinnamon – Ceylon variety (Add 1 tsp. to food/coffee/tea per day)

Take immediately after surgery:

- Multi-vitamin (Take as directed.)
- Vitamin D3 (5,000 IU/day)
- Vitamin K2 (80-120 mcg/day)
- L-Thiamine (100 mg: 1 in the afternoon and 1 before sleep)
- Relora (250 mg: 1 tablet three times/day)
- CoQ-10 – Ubiquinol form (200 mg: 1 tablet/day)
- Methylated B-12 (1,000 mg: 1 tablet/day)
- Quercetin (500-2000 mg/day)
- L-Glutamine (5-10 g/day)
- L-Citrulline (2-6 g/day)
- Probiotic (Look for a supplement containing at least four strains of bacteria)
- Curcumin (with piperine or in a form that increases bio-availability)
- Arnica
- Bromelain
- Cinnamon – Ceylon variety (Add 1 tsp. to food/coffee/tea per day)

Once cleared by your treating physician, take the following additional supplements:

- Kyolic garlic (1 tablet three times/day)
- Omega-3 fatty acids (1-2 g/day)
- Milk Thistle (140 mg: 3 times/day)

As you've probably guessed, all supplements are not created equal.

Two factors that you need to consider when choosing a supplement are the manufacturer and the specific form of the supplement.

Keep in mind these key points when choosing between various forms and manufacturers:

- **Multi-vitamin:** You don't need to spend a fortune to get good quality, but you do need to venture beyond the drugstore brands. Make sure that your multi-vitamin contains a broad base of micronutrients, including many of those cited in the previous chapter. Most of the formulas commercially available are woefully lacking in several key vitamins and minerals (such as Vitamin B12/D3/K2), so you will need to add these to your pre- and post-surgical regimens.
- **CoQ-10:** This area is a little controversial, but it looks as if the Ubiquinol form is more readily absorbed than Ubiquinone.
- **Methylated B-12:** Some people lack the enzyme responsible for actively methylating Vitamin B12, and so are not able to harness its power as effectively. By choosing the activated methylated form, you ensure that your body will be able to actually use it.
- **Probiotic:** This is another area in which you want to purchase a good-quality supplement. Look for a supplement containing at least 5 strains of bacteria and at least 1 billion CFUs (colony-forming units). Many excellent brands do not require refrigeration, which makes it much easier for them to be stored and transported.
- **Curcumin:** Bioavailability is issues with curcumin, so to maximize absorption, make sure that the preparation you buy either contains piperine (a black pepper derivative) or is processed into a form that maximizes bioavailability.

- **Cinnamon:** Always look for Ceylon cinnamon. While all forms of cinnamon contain levels of coumarin (a liver toxin), the Ceylon form contains the lowest levels and is thus one of the safest. Also, don't overdo it on cinnamon. Most physicians recommend ingesting no more than about a teaspoon per day. This should help with blood-sugar control and can also be a tasty perk of whatever you are eating.
- **L-Citrulline:** Increased production of the amino acid L-arginine has been shown to have positive effects on the preservation of lean muscle mass. The issue with direct supplementation of L-arginine itself is that your body will actually up-regulate the enzyme arginase that is responsible for the breakdown of this amino acid when levels increase. To get around this and boost levels, we can supplement with L-citrulline, which is then converted in the body to L-arginine, but without the triggering of the arginase enzyme.
- **Arnica/Bromelain:** I generally recommend a standardized preparation of arnica and bromelain following surgery, which is why no suggested dosage is provided. Although the literature is not definitive with respect to dosing and efficacy, I have personally recommended and used this combination in all of my surgical patients for over a decade with no identifiable side effects.
- **Omega-3 Fatty Acids:** Research into the use of fish oils has covered a very broad range of dosing, so the recommended dose here is on the lower side. Because of the potential for increased bleeding associated with these oils, I suggest starting out low and working with your surgeon to adjust accordingly. When it comes to any marine-sourced supplement, make sure that the product is guaranteed to be free of PCBs and mercury and is pharmaceutical-grade.

One of the most frustrating aspects of writing this book was that while a vast amount of research has gone into evaluating pharmaceutical drugs, far less has gone into evaluating natural remedies for healing and their appropriate dosing.

My hope is that by educating both consumers and medical professionals of the need for this emphasis, more attention will be given to this very important topic.

While drugs are important, so also are preventative methods that can potentially stave off the need for drugs. Therein lies the rub and the potential conflict: At the present time, there is far less emphasis on adequate preparation than there is on treating complications once they occur. As physicians, we should be trained from an early stage to identify nutritional deficiencies and reverse them before they do harm. Given the growing interest from our patients themselves, the movement towards preventative and restorative medicine will undoubtedly continue to grow, and forward-thinking practitioners will continue to shed light on a new direction in medicine that will ultimately prove to be far more helpful to our patients than what we are currently offering. It will be this new paradigm and new thinking that will eventually change the face and the practice of medicine itself.

The Importance of Laboratory Testing

"Nutrition can be compared with a chain in which all essential items are separate links. We know what happens if one link of a chain is weak or is missing. The whole chain falls apart."
- **Patrick Wright, PhD**

Getting ready for surgery can be daunting for even the most organized person. In the days and weeks leading up to the big day, you are nervous, and your only thought is the hope that everything goes smoothly and that you recover as quickly as possible. You are not thinking about how best to prepare.

You just want to get through the procedure unscathed and in one piece. What you are going to eat after may not even have hit your mind and may seem to be of little importance to you, but it should be.

What you eat in the weeks leading up to your surgery and what you eat in the weeks to follow can play a huge role in how you heal. Think about the racecar. You wouldn't race the car without taking the time to make sure that everything is in order and that all its working parts are running smoothly. If you would pay this much attention to a car, why in the world would you jump into surgery without adequately preparing your body? Unfortunately, that is usually what happens. The simple fact that you may not be adequately prepared from a nutritional standpoint may mean the difference between a speedy recovery and one that is plagued with complications and delayed healing.

Preparation for surgery should begin weeks before the actual event. During this time, a few simple steps can mean all the difference in the world in terms of your outcome and the ease of your recovery. Do you really want to figure out meals when you're doped up on pain medications?

Of course not. But this is the way that most of us approach surgery. We focus on the procedure and not on the myriad details surrounding it.

We're not to blame. Considering the amount of information that physicians give you before surgery, it is a wonder that you retain anything at all.

Now that you appreciate the importance of surgical nutrition, how can you best prepare?

To get started, you need to determine how nutritionally fit you really are. To do this, look at a few basic labs.

Remember the racecar analogy? To determine if it is race ready, mechanics begin by looking under the hood and examining the engine. By checking a few key areas, you and your doctor can do the same.

Begin by looking at the following levels. Here's why:

- **Complete Blood Count ("CBC")**
  - o This panel consists of the following labs:
    - *White blood count (WBC)*
      - This tells you if you potentially have an undiagnosed infection, as your WBC tends to rise in the presence of infection.
    - *White blood cell types (WBC differential)*
      - Now that you know the number of WBCs, this test tells you the type of cells contained in that number.
    - *Red blood cell count (RBC count)*
      - Red cells carry oxygen to your tissues, which is critical, not only under normal conditions, but especially during the healing period.

- Too high a number and your blood is too thick. This can lead to slugging and potential blockage of your smaller blood vessels.
- Too low a number, and you may potentially be anemic. This puts the body under increased stress during periods of increased demand (e.g., exercise, healing, etc.).

- *Hematocrit (HCT or Crit)*
  - This test measures the amount of volume that your red blood cells take up in your blood. As such, this test is a very good indicator of anemia.*Hemoglobin (HGB)*
  - The hemoglobin molecule fills red blood cells and is responsible for the actual carrying of oxygen to your tissues. Too little hemoglobin and the local tissue is effectively robbed of oxygen.

- *Red blood cell indices*
  - This test looks at three things: MCV (mean corpuscular volume), MCH (mean corpuscular hemoglobin), and MCHC (mean corpuscular hemoglobin concentration).
  - Your doctor can use these numbers to determine whether you are anemic and which type of anemia you may have.

- *Platelet count*
  - Platelets are essential for clotting, which you will need during surgery.

- Too low a number, and you may have difficulty forming clots, and may bleed more during surgery.
- Too high a number, and you may have an increased tendency to form clots where you don't want them.

- *Mean platelet volume (MPV)*
  - Abnormal numbers may suggest the potential for a clotting issue both during and after your surgery.

- **Basic Metabolic Profile (BMP)**
  - *Blood urea nitrogen (BUN)*
    - This test measures the amount of nitrogen that comes from the waste product urea as protein is broken down within your body.
    - Too high a level may indicate that your kidneys are not functioning properly and may require adjustment of certain medications given to you during and after your surgery.

  - *Creatinine*
    - This test is for the efficiency of your kidneys and their ability to filter waste.
    - Too high a level may indicate that your kidneys are not functioning properly and may require adjustment of certain medications given to you both during and after your surgery.

- *Calcium*
    - ☐ This is a very important electrolyte and mineral responsible for cellular functions.
    - ☐ Levels that are either too high or too low may indicate that something is not functioning properly to maintain this delicate balance.
- *Carbon dioxide*
    - ☐ CO2 is essentially a waste product from metabolism.
    - ☐ Levels that are either too high or too low may indicate that something is not functioning properly to maintain this delicate balance.
- *Chloride*
    - ☐ This is a very important electrolyte and mineral responsible for cellular functions.
    - ☐ Levels that are either too high or too low may indicate that something is not functioning properly to maintain this delicate balance.
- *Glucose*
    - ☐ This measures the sugar level in your blood. Too high, and you may be diabetic or heading in that direction.
    - ☐ Recent studies have shown a correlation between wound-healing complications after surgery and persistent elevation of blood glucose.

- *Potassium*
    - ☐ This is a very important electrolyte and mineral responsible for cellular functions.
    - ☐ Levels that are either too high or too low may indicate that something is not functioning properly to maintain this delicate balance.
- *Sodium*
    - ☐ This is a very important electrolyte and mineral responsible for cellular functions.
    - ☐ Levels that are either too high or too low may indicate that something is not functioning properly to maintain this delicate balance.
- *Fasting Blood Glucose*
    - ☐ How your body handles glucose can be a very powerful indicator of how your body will be able to heal. Several studies have directly shown an increase in wound-healing complications with persistently elevated blood-sugar levels.
    - ☐ Along with HgbA1C level, your doctor can also determine your risk for insulin resistance and manage accordingly.

- *Ferritin*
  - ☐ Iron is stored within the protein ferritin, so ferritin levels are a direct indication of your body's total iron storage capacity.
  - ☐ Too high, and you could be sitting on toxic levels of iron, which can harm your liver and other organs. Too low, and you may experience signs and symptoms of anemia, as well as delayed wound-healing.
- *Retinol Binding Protein (RBP)*
  - ☐ RBP is important as the carrier for Vitamin A within your body.
  - ☐ It is also used to correlate overall visceral protein mass. Low levels may suggest a protein deficiency and thus an increased potential for delayed healing.
- *Albumin*
  - ☐ Albumin is a protein made in the liver and released into the bloodstream.
  - ☐ Binding and transport of many small molecules in the blood, such as bilirubin, calcium, and magnesium, as well as many drugs
  - ☐ Maintenance of colloid osmotic pressure
  - ☐ Free radical scavenging
  - ☐ Acid-base balance
  - ☐ Pro- and anti-coagulator effects (inhibits platelet aggregation, enhances the inhibition of factor Xa by antithrombin III)

- ☐ Maintenance of optimal vascular permeability
- ☐ Albumin has a half-life of around 20 days, so it represents a more chronic picture of your overall protein balance.
- *Pre-Albumin*
  - ☐ This is a protein that is made in the liver and released into the blood. Its role is to carry certain hormones that regulate how your body uses energy, in addition to carrying other substances through your body.
  - ☐ Low pre-albumin levels may suggest malnutrition related to a poor diet and may potentially point to an increased risk for wound healing following your surgery.
  - ☐ Albumin has a half-life of only two to three days, so it represents a more acute picture of your overall protein balance.
- *Vitamin D*
  - ☐ Although it is called a vitamin, many physicians now regard this as a pro-hormone because of its many effects through the body.
  - ☐ Unfortunately, because of a growing trend towards sun avoidance, many of us are continuously running in the red when it comes to low Vitamin D levels.

- Although your mother may have told you to drink your milk to increase Vitamin D levels, this is actually a very inefficient way to increase stores. Oral supplements along with Vitamin K2, is generally recommended.

- *Hemoglobin A1C*
  - Once reserved just for diabetics, this lab measures your average blood sugar levels for the past two to three months.
  - More specifically, it identifies what percentage of your hemoglobin (the protein in your blood that carries oxygen) is coated with sugar (glycated).
  - Recent studies have demonstrated an increased risk for wound-healing complications associated with chronically elevated blood-sugar levels, so an adjustment here may potentially improve your chances for optimal wound healing.

Your doctor may recommend additional labs, or may not recommend any labs at all, depending upon the type of surgery being performed and your overall health. While some doctors may question the efficacy of these labs, they are quick and easy safeguards that will potentially point out any pitfalls and deficiencies before surgery that can be easily corrected simply by adjusting your diet or adding a few over-the-counter supplements. This is your life; do you really want to jump into surgery and hope that you recover smoothly? I didn't think so.

...he following labs at least two to four weeks ...before your surgery, and again two weeks after surgery, to ensure that you have the optimal chance for healing:

- ☐ Complete blood count (CBC)
- ☐ Basic metabolic profile (BMP)
- ☐ Albumin/Pre-albumin
- ☐ Fasting blood glucose
- ☐ Ferritin
- ☐ Retinol binding protein (RBP)
- ☐ Vitamin D
- ☐ Hemoglobin A1C

Your Recipes for Success

"Don't eat anything your great-great-grandmother wouldn't recognize as food. There are a great many food-like items in the supermarket your ancestors wouldn't recognize as foods...stay away from these."
- Michael Pollan
American author, journalist, activist, and professor of journalism at the UC Berkeley Graduate School of Journalism

Now that you appreciate the importance of surgical nutrition, let's look at options to help you heal better, faster, and more effortlessly following your surgery. I encourage you to review the chapters on individual macro/micronutrients first so that you understand why specific ingredients are being incorporated.

Although I provided a veritable laundry list of potential aids for healing, I don't expect you to use all of these ingredients and would actually encourage you not to so that you can keep everything as simple as possible. Getting ready for surgery is a huge undertaking, and the last thing you need is more complexity. With that in mind, let's take a look at a few options.

In reviewing the following recipes, work with your treating physician to determine whether there are any ingredients that should not be included and whether or not these would interfere with any medications or any dietary restrictions you will have both before and after your surgery.
Many patients have difficulty consuming solid foods after surgery, so we will emphasize a more liquid-based diet so that you are actually able to consume them. Many of my own patients find that they enjoy these recipes so much that they continue to make them long after their surgeries. These are all very healthy, and, more importantly, they taste good!

My first quick tip is a product that I feel is essential to good health and one that I use on a daily basis.

For those of you who, like me, are old enough to remember the cheesy commercials, this product is Vitamix®. Before I begin, let me emphasize that I have no financial relationship with the company whatsoever. I own three devices and keep them at my home, at my fiancé's home, and at my office, and use them to make a variety of healthy foods. While I strongly urge you to buy one to use for good health in general, I also think they are an excellent resource for meal production around the time of surgery.

Many of my patients have little appetite following surgery, and may not feel like eating solid foods, but they don't want to swill down a disgusting protein shake that tastes awful and leaves their mouth with that chalky residue. Voilà, Vitamix®! In a matter of minutes, they can whip up a delicious shake that is good for them.

Like most people, before buying a Vitamix®, I was trying hard to get enough vegetables in my diet and, quite frankly, was not doing a very good job. The prep was killing me, and I did not have enough time to sit and eat the volume that I was supposed to. Now, I simply create a protein base for my shakes (usually whey powder) and add my favorite veggies, fruit, healthy fat source, and any additional flavorings. I can whip up a drink in five minutes or fewer.

You can easily incorporate shakes into your post-surgical meal plan by simply prepping the ingredients and placing them in a sealable plastic bag or reusable container and placing them in the freezer.
When you're ready, simply pull out your protein powder, add the pre-assembled ingredients, and you're good to go.

SOUPS

Bone Broth Stock

- ☐ 3 pounds beef marrow bones (only from a high-quality beef source – e.g., grass-fed beef)
- ☐ Optional: Chicken feet or necks (This will further increase the collagen content of your broth.)
- ☐ Optional: Ox tail (This will definitely enhance the rich flavor of the overall broth.)
- ☐ 2 tbsp. apple cider vinegar
- ☐ Water (to cover)
- ☐ 3 stalks celery, chopped into 3 pieces
- ☐ 3 carrots, peeled and chopped into 2 pieces
- ☐ 1 yellow onion, chopped into 4 pieces
- ☐ 3 bay leaves
- ☐ 3 cloves garlic (preferably roasted)
- ☐ 1 tbsp. peppercorns (black or mixed)

Begin by placing the bones on a cooking sheet in an oven pre-heated to 350 degrees Fahrenheit for 30 minutes. Once braised, remove the bones, place them in a large soup pan or slow cooker, and cover with water (filtered if you prefer). Let the bones cool for 30 minutes.

Add the celery, carrots, onion, bay leaves, garlic, and peppercorns. Cover with any additional water as needed. Bring to a boil, cover, and reduce heat to simmer for 48 hours.

During cooking, stir as needed (maybe every 6 hours or so), and add water to cover as necessary. If you leave the pot uncovered, you will need to add water more frequently, as the water boils off.
I find it much easier to cover the pot at least partially to avoid this. This will determine how thick the final stock is.

Cook the stock down for 48 hours. Strain off all solids and let cool. Place in the refrigerator overnight. Once cooled, the fat will have congealed on the top. Using a slotted spoon or spatula, remove this fat and discard.

Ladle the remaining fluid into small reusable containers or ice cube trays and place in the freezer. The stock can be stored for months and easily heated up to make soup. The stock cubes can be removed from the trays (once frozen), placed in a re-sealable bag, and used for smaller portion sizes.

To use the stock, simply remove from the freezer, and place the reusable container under warm water until the frozen stock can be easily transferred into a soup pot. Add water to adjust desired consistency and flavor by adding your choice of meat, vegetables, spices, and salt.

You can also use the stock as a tasty drink. Simply place 2-4 frozen cubes in a microwave coffee mug, and warm. The broth is delicious, nutritious, and easy on your stomach. Add salt to flavor, but please use sparingly. The more salt you consume, the more you will swell!

Chicken Soup

- ☐ 1 kosher or free-range chicken
- ☐ Water
- ☐ 1 tbsp. virgin olive oil
- ☐ 5 celery stalks, coarsely chopped
- ☐ 5 carrots, peeled and coarsely chopped
- ☐ 1 yellow onion, finely chopped
- ☐ 3 cloves garlic, finely chopped
- ☐ 1 tsp. thyme
- ☐ 3 bay leaves
- ☐ ½-1 tsp. black pepper
- ☐ 1 cup white wine
- ☐ Sea salt (to flavor as needed)

Wash chicken (removing any organs, as necessary), then place on a cooking sheet. Brush lightly with oil, and bake at 375 degrees Fahrenheit for 20-25 minutes until the skin begins to turn a light golden brown.

Remove from oven, and allow the chicken to cool for about 10-15 minutes. Place in a large stockpot, cover with water and bring to a boil. Once boiling, turn down the heat, and simmer for up to 4 hours. Remove chicken, and allow it to cool.

Once cooled, remove all meat, and place in a separate dish. Return the bones, skin, and remaining fat to the same pot, and cover with water. Bring to a boil, and then continue to simmer.

In a separate pot, add the olive oil, celery, carrots, onion, and garlic, and sweat the vegetables on medium heat until they turn translucent (about 10 minutes). Add thyme, bay leaves, white wine, and pepper. Add chicken meat. Cover with water as needed. Bring to a boil, and then reduce to simmer uncovered until fluid is reduced by about ½ of its original volume.

Once the other pot (water/chicken bones, skin, and fat) has simmered for about 3 hours, strain all solids from this pot, and add the fluid to the pot containing the vegetables and meat. Continue cooking at a simmer for about 30 minutes. Salt to taste.

This chicken soup can be frozen in reusable containers and used as needed. In addition, I often add wild rice to the soup to create a heartier meal and bump up the protein content.

Macro-Nutrient Balanced Protein Smoothies

I am a huge fan of protein shakes, not only for my surgical patients, but also for me. I consume one to two shakes a day and use them to balance out my daily dietary intake quickly and simply with healthy ingredients that I might not ingest with my other meals.

Following surgery, protein shakes can be lifesavers! Think about it: You have just had surgery, you do not really feel like eating solid food, and you may not have much of an appetite. Most protein shake supplements alone taste horrible; trust me, I've tried them! They also tend to cost way more than the price of simply making a delicious shake yourself, choosing ingredients that you actually like and the taste that you actually want.

To help balance dietary intake, it's best to combine ingredients from all three of the major macronutrients (carbohydrates/proteins/fats) and then add additional ingredients (herbs, spices, and other flavorings) as you see fit. I have outlined several choices to make it easy for you to create these shakes quickly and simply. To make it even easier, we encourage you to prep out the raw ingredients before your surgery and place them in a freezer bag or reusable container and put it into the freezer. Once you need them, simply take them out, and add them to your liquid base. Pretty easy!

Protein + Fat + Carb + Liquid + Other = Delicious Shake
To get started, let's talk about the basics.

Liquid base +/- some healthy carbs to approximately 8-14 ounces of liquid (based on thickness preference):

- ☐ Purified water; *freshly* juiced juice (greens/lemon/apple juice); unsweetened tea(s); and/or unsweetened almond, coconut, flax, and/or hazelnut milk *[handwritten: Use (chocolate) Pansley protein powder or pumpkin seed powder]*

Protein source (preferably hypoallergenic, amino-acid complete protein powder[s]. Try to add around 20-30 grams of protein/shake:

- [ ] Pea, rice, pumpkin seed, and/or sacha inchi protein powders
- [ ] **Or** a combination of *at least* 2 of these protein powders
- [ ] **Or** whey protein (if not sensitive or allergic to dairy products)

The carbohydrate portion of the smoothie, watch calories, as they can add up pretty easily with a small amount of carbs (for example, a few whole pieces of fruit). Therefore, if you intend to consume two or more smoothies per day as part of your meal plan, try to keep the carbohydrate portion to about 1/2 of (or) equal to (1:1 ratio) the protein portion of the smoothie.

- [ ] For example: Blueberries (1/2 cup) *[handwritten: 1/4 cup]* and Apple (1/2) – one day

And

- [ ] Raspberries (1/2 cup) and banana (1/2 only) – on another day or with another protein smoothie

Plus….

- [ ] **BEST**: Leafy greens and/or cruciferous veggies (e.g., Mixed greens, kale, spinach, bok choy, broccoli, yellow summer squash, etc.—generally use approximately 1/2 to 1 cup, but feel free to splurge and use a little more, since all of these carbohydrate sources are very low glycemic in addition to being very cleansing to your liver and other tissues.)
- [ ] See the carbohydrate listing of BEST/OKAY/AVOID carbohydrates for more information on which ones to use and which ones to avoid.

Fats

- [ ] Best: Extra-virgin olive oil, extra-virgin coconut oil (1 tbsp./smoothie), or avocado oil (approximately 1/3 of a Haas avocado/smoothie)
- [ ] Almond, pumpkin, hazelnut, or macadamia nut butter (approximately 1-2 tbsp./smoothie) *not pb or cashew*

Fiber

- [ ] Flax and/or chia-seed powder (ground and ideally *sprouted*)— (1 tbsp./smoothie) for increased fiber and protein content and to feel satiated longer
- [ ] You will also receive extra fiber simply by choosing from the BEST and OKAY carbohydrate sources.

No (or) low-glycemic natural sweetener alternatives (optional):

- [ ] Organic stevia (a non-blood-sugar/non-insulin-inducing, *natural* sweetener)—Add to taste, and use as you would sprinkle pepper on food.
- [ ] Top-tasting and -priced products:
100% pure, powdered version by NOW® Foods or Liquid, *non-alcoholic* version by SweetLeaf®, which comes in fantastic, really potent flavors, (e.g., chocolate, vanilla, English toffee, etc.)
Coconut sugar (in moderation)
Lo Han (in moderation)
Xylitol (in moderation)

Spices/Flavorings (optional):

- [ ] Cinnamon – Very good for balancing blood sugar
- [ ] Cloves
- [ ] Nutmeg
- [ ] Raw cacao or cocoa powder (multiple health benefits)

- ☐ Ginger root
- ☐ Turmeric

Supplements

While there are a number of supplements that you can take both before and after your surgery, you are most likely going to be taking a number of medications, so the goal is to keep your list as simple as possible. I would suggest the following regimen:

Before Surgery

- ☐ Multi-vitamin (preferably from a natural source)
- ☐ L-Citrulline (1,000 mg: Up to 6,000 mg/day)
- ☐ CoQ-10 (100 mg: 1 tablet/day)
- ☐ Methylated B-12 (1,000 mg: 1 tablet/day)
- ☐ Prebiotic (FOS/Inulin)
- ☐ Probiotic (Look for a supplement containing at least four strains of bacteria)
- ☐ L-Theanine (100 mg: 1 in the afternoon and 1 before sleep)
- ☐ Relora (250 mg: 1 tablet three times/day)

After Surgery

- ☐ Multi-vitamin (preferably from a natural source)
- ☐ L-Glutamine (5,000 mg/day: tablet or powder)
- ☐ L-Citrulline (1,000 mg: Up to 6000 mg/day)
- ☐ CoQ-10 (100 mg: 1 tablet/day)
- ☐ Methylated B-12 (1,000 mg: 1 tablet/day)
- ☐ Prebiotic (FOS/Inulin)
- ☐ Probiotic (Look for a supplement containing at least four strains of bacteria)
- ☐ L-Thiamine (100 mg: 1 in the afternoon and 1 before sleep)
  Relora (250 mg: 1 tablet three times/day)

Once cleared by your treating physician, you can add the following supplements:

☐ Kyolic garlic (1 tablet three times/day)
☐ Omega-3 fatty acids (1-2 g/day)

Suggested Ingredients

To emphasize as healthy a meal as possible, please use only quality ingredients. Remember, your body is healing and needs good stuff, not a lot of pesticides, hormones, and other additives. When choosing ingredients, I recommend the following:

Vegetables

☐ Preferably organic

Berries

☐ Preferably organic
☐ No sugar added

Meats

☐ Free-range/kosher/chicken/turkey
☐ Grass-fed beef and beef bones

Protein Powders

☐ Animal-based proteins:
- Whey protein isolate/concentrate
- Egg white protein concentrate
- Cricket protein concentrate
- Collagen peptides

Ideally, look for brands that contain organically derived proteins with no or low glycemic, naturally derived/extracted flavorings and/or sweeteners (e.g., organic stevia powder, flavored organic stevia liquid drops, Lo Han extract powder, or xylitol powder), and with no artificial or low-quality added ingredients that can negatively affect your health and even your weight! You simply don't need them. Flavor is your choice!

☐ **Vegetable-Based Proteins:**

- Brown rice protein concentrate
- Pea protein isolate
- Pumpkin seed protein concentrate
- Sacha inchi seed protein concentrate

*For optimal amino acid ratio balance and protein quality, look for a combination protein product with some (or) all of the latest, high-quality, cold-processed vegetable proteins listed above.

Great for vegans. deally look for brands that contain organically derived proteins with no or low glycemic, naturally derived/extracted flavorings and/or sweeteners (e.g., organic stevia, Lo Han extract powder, or xylitol powder) and with no artificial or low-quality, added ingredients that may negatively affect your health and even your weight! You simply don't need them. Flavor is your choice!

AVOID soy isolate protein powders. This is not a high-quality protein. Bloating and gas is common and obviously not what you want to occur either before or after your surgery. It potentially causes dangerous hormone imbalances in women as well as in men!

Under normal conditions, your body requires quality ingredients to help it run efficiently.

During times of stress or trauma (such as surgery), this need increases and become even more important. If you want to heal and heal well, you need to do a little work, but this work need not be time-consuming. The benefits in terms of quality of healing, energy levels, and overall feeling of wellness will far surpass your expectations.

In the next section we will focus on several healing hacks, which will help speed your time to recovery and make the overall process much more tolerable.

Hacking Your Healing: Optimizing the Mind-Body Connection

"When you see the Golden Arches you are probably on the road to the Pearly Gates."
- William Catelli, MD (Director, Framingham Heart Study)

Healing is an individual experience and obviously varies from person to person, based not only on the type of procedure being performed but also on how you individually handle discomfort. But healing doesn't need to be hard.

As a surgeon, I've put together a number of tips and tricks over the years that I have passed down to my patients in an effort to make their recoveries as smooth and as optimized as possible. I am sharing them now with you!

To better organize this list, I've broken them down into two main categories: MIND and BODY.

The MIND

Surgery and the healing period immediately following it can be stressful. Stress is not helpful to our bodies. The more you calm your mind before and after surgery, the more pleasant the overall experience will be for you and potentially the better you will heal. Many patients develop mind monkey or monkey mind (from Chinese *Xin yuan* and Sino-Japanese "heart-/mind-monkey"). This is a Buddhist term meaning "unsettled; restless; capricious; whimsical; fanciful; inconstant; confused; indecisive; uncontrollable". To help reduce anxiety both before and after your procedure, there are several practices we have found to be helpful and that we are beginning to recommend to our patients.

Stress triggers the hormone cortisol, which can have negative effects not only on how you heal, but also on your overall health. Tempering the effects of cortisol may potentially lead to a smoother recovery and to improved overall health.

To reduce stress and focus your mind, we suggest the following options:

BEFORE SURGERY

- **Aromatherapy:** The use of specific scented oils can be a very effective way to reduce stress and focus the mind during the perioperative period. The following aromatherapy regimens were provided by my good friend and board-certified anesthesiologist **Dr. Nancy Thurman** for use before and after surgery. The good news is that they do not interfere with surgery itself or any medications you may receive while under anesthesia. I can personally attest to their benefit and receive a tremendous amount of positive feedback from my own patients who undergo anesthesia with Dr. Thurman and who feel much calmer and more relaxed prior to induction.

  Studies have shown that how you go to sleep before surgery plays a huge role in how you wake up after surgery.

  Use **lavender** to help you sleep the night before or to help ease anxiety the morning of surgery. Lavender is especially helpful if used in bath water, in lotions and moisturizers for the face and body, or as mists. Spraying lavender on your pillow at night can help with insomnia. I give patients a little lavender mixed with witch hazel the morning of surgery to ease nervousness.

  "Rose and geranium are floral aromatherapies that can help focus your mind before or after surgery."

*"**Citrus (orange, lime, lemon, lemon eucalyptus, tangerine, and grapefruit)** are aromas that can be energizing and detoxifying. I recommend using these aromatherapies to help you wake up and to get the anesthesia out of your system. Orange mixes well with lavender."*

*"**Peppermint and spearmint** are both excellent for patients in the recovery room for controlling nausea and vomiting. I use a mixture of these two mints in mild carrier oil such as grape seed oil under the patient's nose when they come out of anesthesia. Mints wake you up, help with nausea, and moreover relieve headaches associated with anesthesia."*

*"**Ginger** is also an excellent anti-nausea aromatherapy regimen. Its aroma is less pungent than the mints, so it can be used to dilute down the mint if needed."*

"My recovery room mixture includes lavender, ginger, peppermint, and spearmint. Mix a few drops of each in carrier oil such as grape seed oil, almond oil, or apricot seed oil. You can pick and choose each amount of the essential oils to your aromatherapy tastes for a nicer recovery room experience."

- **Guided meditation/focused breathing:** Controlling how you breathe can play a huge role in your heart rate and release of excitatory a hormone called catecholamine. In turn, this can help regulate levels of the stress hormone cortisol. Deep breathing can evoke a relaxation response and actually slow your heartbeat and lower your blood pressure.

  To practice focused breathing, simply find a quiet, comfortable place to either sit or lie down. Begin by taking a normal breath. Then take a deeper breath by inhaling slowly through your nose while allowing your chest and lower belly to rise as you fill your lungs.

Allow your abdomen to expand fully. Now, release your breath slowly through your mouth, and repeat.

We encourage our patients to begin a program of meditation/focused breathing in the weeks leading up to their surgeries so that this becomes a natural part of their daily regimen. Once you are done with surgery and comfortable with a specific program, you can utilize its benefits to calm your nerves and focus on optimal healing.

To make this as easy as possible, we recommend using one of the many apps available on either the iPhone or Android. Many of these offer some form of trial membership or introductory viewing, so you can identify which specific program works best for you. Here are a few that I enjoyed:

- Calm.com
- Buddhify 2
- Headspace
- Omvana
- Simply Being
- Breathe Sync
- Tactical Breather
- Breathe2Relax

- **Binaural beats therapy (BBT):** By playing the two different tones (one in each ear) through headphones, researchers have found that your central nervous system will actually produce a composite signal with a frequency resulting from the difference of the two frequencies. This new tone has been thought to cause hemispheric synchronization and effectively guide the brain into a specific brain wave frequency. The frequency of 4 Hz (delta-theta rhythm) is considered by most researchers to favor the state of calm and relaxation.

To examine the effects of BBT on surgical patients, researchers at Chiang Mai University in Thailand divided elderly patients undergoing cataract surgery (often performed under local anesthesia alone) into groups of 47. The first group listened to binaural beats and music coupled with natural noises, the second group listened to music and natural noises alone, and the third group listened to nothing at all. Using the STAI (State Trait Anxiety Inventory) scale, researchers found that the BBT group demonstrated a significant decrease in anxiety and systolic blood pressure compared to those patients listening to nothing at all. There was a slight reduction in the same parameters for the music group, as well. According to researcher **Dr. Pornattana Vichitvejpaisal**, *"Our study shows significant emotional and physiological benefits from adding binaural beats to music therapy for cataract surgery patients. This provides a simple, inexpensive way to improve patients' health outcomes and satisfaction with their care."* Findings of this preliminary study were recently presented at the annual meeting of the American Academy of Ophthalmology.

I have personally used BBT for relaxation and have found it to be very effective for promoting states of relaxation. I would recommend the following free apps:

- Binaural Beats
- Binaural – Pure Binaural Beats
- Beyond Meditation Binaural Beats

- **Biofeedback:** While the origin of biofeedback can be traced as far back as the early Hindus and Buddhists, it didn't morph into its more contemporary form until just after World War II.

Biofeedback works by attaching various instruments to your body to directly measure physiological activity, such as brain waves, heart rate, body temperature, respiratory rate, and muscle tension. These devices allow you to see real-time measurements and changes in specific vitals.

With this feedback, you can potentially make changes to these vitals simply by adjusting your breathing and depth of relaxation.

The use of biofeedback programs to actively monitor and modulate vital signs has become very popular over the last few years as more Americans look for ways to reduce their stress. Before and after surgery, biofeedback can be especially helpful in not only regulating specific vitals, but also in identifying how much you are stressed

Again, to make this as easy as possible, we recommend a number of available iPhone and Android apps. Many of these will monitor vitals using your camera function. Others require the purchase of separate monitoring modalities that, in my mind, are actually far more effective at truly identifying correct vitals, as well as brainwave activity.

Consider the following options:

- Muse:

    - Headset + app (iPhone/Android)

- Bio Zen:

    - Free app (Android) + Bluetooth-enabled biosensors (Zephyr BioHarness measures heart rate, respiration, and skin temperature; MindWave™ Mobile measures brainwave activity).
    - Sensors measure EEG (brain wave activity), EMG (muscle tension), skin temperature, respiratory rate, and ECG (heart rate variability).

- BioZen also has a meditation feature, which allows users to manipulate an image on their smartphone screen with their mind and heart rate activity.

  o emWave2:

  - Device + computer program
  - Measures heart rate variability
  - Using a pulse rate monitor, heart rate variability can be monitored and adjusted to reach a state of coherence.

- **Yoga:** It seems that every day another study supports the many health benefits of yoga. Many people who practice yoga refer to it as a "moving meditation". Before surgery, establishing a practice of yoga can help you focus your mind and relieve stress; after surgery it can do the same. Depending on the type of surgery you will undergo, be sure to receive clearance from your surgeon before resuming yoga (after surgery). Many of my patients are avid practitioners and generally return to their practices within five to six weeks of their procedures.
- **Dr. Google:** This is a tough one and a double-edged sword. While more and more people use the Internet to research various health conditions, many of the sites that they use are either outdated, inaccurate, or simply wrong.

If you do decide to learn more about your condition, your surgery, and what to expect, at least use a source that is credible. I recommend the following sites to my patients and to you:

- WebMD® (www.webmd.com)
- eMedicineHealth (www.emedicinehealth.com)

- The Cleveland Clinic Health Information Center (http://my.clevelandclinic.org/health)
- Mayo Clinic (www.mayoclinic.com)
- Healthfinder.gov (www.healthfinder.gov)
- Net Wellness® (www.netwellness.org)
- MedlinePlus® (www.medlineplus.gov)

RIGHT BEFORE SURGERY

- **Aromatherapy:** I have received a ton of positive feedback from my patients regarding our use of aromatherapy on the day of surgery. Hats off to Dr. Thurman for introducing me to this amazing way to keep my patients focused and relaxed before and after their procedures. (See above)
- **Music therapy:** A number of studies have confirmed the beneficial effects of music not only before surgery but also during the actual procedure.

The Lancet recently featured a meta-analysis of 72 randomized trials of perioperative music, reported by Jenny Hole and colleagues, showing that music was associated with modest reductions in patient-reported postoperative pain and anxiety, reduced analgesia use, and increased patient satisfaction ("Music as an aid for postoperative recovery in adults: a systematic review and meta-analysis." **Jenny Hole, MBBS, Martin Hirsch, MBBS, Elizabeth Ball**, PhD, and **Catherine Meads, PhD**; Published online August 12, 2015).

- **Guided meditation/focused breathing:** See above
- **Biofeedback:** See above
- **Dr. Google:** See above.

After Surgery

- **Aromatherapy:** See above.
- **Music therapy:** See above.

- **Guided meditation/focused breathing:** See above.
- **Biofeedback:** See above.
- **Dr. Google:** See above.
- **Yoga:** See above.

The BODY

Some things cannot be controlled after surgery, but many things can. To effectively hack your healing, consider the following steps:

- **Healing foods:** In addition to recipes provided in the previous chapter, there are a number of foods and food ingredients that can potentially make your healing period much better:

  o Protein: Supplement with protein before surgery to ensure that you have adequate protein stores and are prepared for the healing period ahead. After surgery, protein is also a necessary macronutrient as the "building block" of a majority of your body's cells.
  Many people do not realize that protein is also a mild diuretic and can actually pull water from your body. During this early healing period, protein may help speed your body's elimination of excess fluids and help reduce your overall swelling.

  o Asparagus: Most fitness professionals appreciate the diuretic effect of asparagus and use it to rid their bodies of excess water before competitions. You can do the same following surgery. Be prepared, however, for that funky smell to your urine. If that is the worst side effect that you encounter, I'd say that the benefit is definitely worth it!

Don't forget that asparagus also contains a number of healthy macro and micronutrients that will help speed healing.

o Flavored water: One of the biggest issues that many of us have with or without surgery is our inability to drink enough water. Following surgery, water intake can be critical as a hydrating agent but also as an agent for flushing unwanted toxins from your body. To make a delicious pitcher of flavored water, simply add your favorite fresh or frozen fruits (and/or vegetables) to a pitcher of filtered water. Whatever ingredients you add to the water will impart their specific flavors to this very healthy (and delicious) drink. My personal favorites include lemon/lime slices, frozen fruit, cucumbers, and fresh mint, but feel free to be creative and add whatever you like to create your own individualized and tasty flavored water!

o Lemon juice: Our bodies prefer to exist in an alkaline state, but many of the foods we eat push them towards the acidic side. To provide balance, I encourage all of my patients (surgical and non-surgical) to drink the juice of half a lemon in water every morning. This drink should then be followed by a full glass of water to flush the acid from your teeth and avoid potential etching. Alkalinizing your body is especially important for anyone consuming high levels of protein, as protein itself tends to push the body's acid-base balance toward the acidic side.

o Pre-made meals: I cannot say enough about the importance of pre-made meals.

Whether these are meals that you have personally prepared and refrigerated/frozen or they are purchased from a healthy source, meals that are ready to go can potentially mean the difference between you eating and you not eating. Pre-made does not include Lean Cuisine and other meals that are full of preservatives and devoid of healthy ingredients. The time you spend preparing a few meals before surgery will pay off in spades when you are sore, tired, and you have no energy left to cook following your surgery. Be careful, though; if you're going to purchase pre-made meals, know the source. Many local businesses are popping up around the country offering prepped meals, but the pure and simple fact is that many of these are just not healthy. Although this may sound crazy, I suggest contacting your local gym rat (i.e., bodybuilder or cross-fit guru) to find out where they buy their meals. In Denver alone, there are several options for healthy meals; it just depends on your tastes and where you live in the city.

- **Lymphatic massage:** Following surgery, your entire body reacts to the trauma. You don't just hold in water and swell around the site of the actual surgery. An effect on your whole body is a normal response and one that is guided not only by inflammatory meditators but also by your hormones themselves. To rid the body of excess fluid, many practitioners (such as myself) use lymphatic massage to help direct excess fluid towards open lymphatic channels for excretion. Before you do this, please get clearance from your surgeon, and locate a trained professional who is experienced specifically in the area of lymphatic massage.

- **Walks**: Believe it or not, this is actually a very powerful tool that you can use to relax and improve your focus following surgery. Walking not only improves circulatory flow (gets your blood pumping and potentially reduces your risk for deep vein thrombosis or DVT); it also can potentially help clear your mind.

Once they are cleared to ambulate (and I clear my patients very early), my patients are instructed to walk outside for brief periods of time (15 to 30 minutes). I truly believe that these walks not only help improve circulation and breathing (which then decreases the risk of pulmonary infections), but that they also help to improve mood. Being trapped in bed or even simply in the house for prolonged periods of time can make anyone go stir-crazy. Trust me...just try it!

I hope these recommendations are helpful, and I look forward to hearing feedback on how they better prepared you for your surgery. Let me know what you think!

What You Need for Optimal Health

"Today, more than 95% of all chronic disease is caused by food choice, toxic food ingredients, nutritional deficiencies, and lack of physical exercise."
- **Mike Adams**

I am a huge proponent of healthy nutrition, not only to help patients achieve optimal wellness, but also as an aid in my patients' recoveries following surgery. But healthy eating is an important topic that many people simply do not understand. When it comes to physicians, most of us have little to no background in nutrition and do not have the interest or the time to properly educate our patients on the foods and supplements they can use to help guide their healing in the right direction.

As a patient, you need to know what will help you heal properly and what will provide you with enough energy. Before surgery, your thoughts are focused on how to manage life during the early healing period; that leaves you with little time to research what you need. While there is a huge amount of information available on nutrition, both on and offline, this information is often confusing and hard to sort out. Let's start with the basics.

All food is composed of nutrients, which can be further broken down into macronutrients and micronutrients. Macronutrients need to be consumed in large amounts and include fats, carbohydrates, proteins, water, and fiber. Micronutrients, which are only needed in much smaller amounts, include vitamins, minerals, herbs, and other important compounds. To guarantee a balanced diet before and after surgery, you need the right nutrients but also in the right amounts.

What your body normally needs may be completely different than what it needs following a stress such as surgery. Your body reacts to the trauma of surgery by changing levels of various hormones to adapt to the shock of the procedure and to initiate healing. It undergoes a tremendous amount of inflammation, depending upon the extent of your surgery and the degree of tissue injury. This is a time when building blocks of repair are important, but so are the various nutrients that help restore your body and reduce inflammation.

Your body's metabolic demands will increase, as will your caloric demands, making what you eat and how much you eat even more critical.

Let's turn our attention to the specific nutrients and their vital roles in the process of healing.

Macronutrients

"It's bizarre that the produce manager is more important to my children's health than the pediatrician."
- Meryl Streep (actress)

As their name implies, macronutrients are necessary in much larger amounts than micronutrients, and they are undoubtedly the nutrients we are most familiar with. This group of nutrients is comprised of several key players, including:

☐ Fats
☐ Carbohydrates
☐ Proteins
☐ Fiber
☐ Water

In the pages we will discuss specifics of each macronutrient, along with recommendations to help improve your overall health and optimize healing.

Fats

If you are American, chances are you have heard about fat. The news may not have all been good, but not all fats are bad! In fact, without fat, your body would be in bad shape, and you could even die.

Your body needs fat for a number of vital functions. Without it, you will have trouble absorbing and maintaining proper levels of fat-soluble vitamins, such as Vitamins A, D, E, and K. Too little Vitamin A, and your eyes suffer, and you develop night blindness. Too little Vitamin K and your blood fails to clot. Low levels of Vitamin D can make your bones brittle and lead to rickets in children and osteomalacia in adults. Vitamin E deficiency, though rare, can lead to muscle weakness and problems with vision. Other global symptoms of fat-soluble vitamin deficiency can lead to dry skin and eczema, in addition to a slew of other skin conditions.

Fat is also an incredibly important energy source. When fat is burned, a total of nine kilocalories/gram is released, which makes fat our most robust source of energy. This quality of fat, along with it being essential for the absorption and storage of fat-soluble vitamins, underscores the importance of this critical nutrient under normal conditions, as well as before and after a surgical procedure.

As a group, fats are described as either "unsaturated" or "saturated," depending upon their chemical structure.

Unsaturated fats differ from saturated fats visually in that unsaturated fats are liquid at room temperature. This type of fat may actually lower cholesterol and so is considered to be a healthier choice of fat. Unsaturated fats can be further broken down into two main groups: mono-unsaturated fats (MUFA) and poly-unsaturated fats (PUFA).

MUFAs (or omega-9 fatty acids) are typically found in avocados; nuts; and specific vegetable oils, such as canola, olive, and peanut oil. They may help lower your LDL (bad) cholesterol, while increasing levels of your HDL (good) cholesterol.

Getting the right amount of unsaturated fat is important so that we obtain the essential fatty acids (EFAs): linoleic (also known as omega-6 fatty acids) and linolenic acids (also known as omega-3 fatty acids in plant form). Linolenic (omega-3) oils are found in plant sources, such as soybean oil, canola oil, walnut oil, flaxseed, and chia seed oil. Because omega-3s have a known anti-platelet effect, many practitioners recommend that you stop using them at least two weeks before surgery and don't start again until you get the green light from your surgeon.

Even this conventional wisdom is now being put to the test. These EFAs are fatty acids that we must ingest. Our bodies require them for good health but cannot synthesize them. In addition, and most importantly, once we ingest the plant form of linolenic acid, our bodies must then convert it to the biologically active forms of omega-3 fatty acids called EPA and DHA. This process, especially as we age, is often difficult to accomplish. Therefore, a more efficient and direct way to achieve optimal levels of EPA and DHA in the body is to consume animal-based, preformed amounts of EPA and DHA. This can easily be accomplished by consuming the highest quality animal sources, such as fish (e.g., wild salmon, wild cod, grass-fed beef, and/or flaxseed-fed chicken eggs), marine sources (e.g., herring, sardines, Pacific oysters, trout, and Atlantic/Pacific mackerel), or by simply taking an EPA/DHA omega-3 fatty acid supplement.

If we do not consume enough omega-6 and omega-3 fatty acids, we are unable to produce a variety of hormones and hormone-like substances that help regulate processes in our kidneys, gut, immune system, bloodstream, and even our brain.

EFA deficiencies can often be seen as any one or more of the following:

- Dry, flaky skin
- Small bumps on the back of your upper arms
- Dandruff or "cradle cap"
- Brittle, cracking fingernails
- Dull fingernails
- Dry eyes
- Vaginal dryness
- Menstrual cramps
- Pre-menstrual breast pain and/or tenderness
- New onset or worsening allergies
- Craving of fatty foods
- Stiff or painful joints

As if that were not enough, very low-fat diets can also produce negative effects on levels of the sex hormones estrogen and testosterone. In women this can dramatically alter menstrual cycles, in addition to weakening bones given estrogen's critical role in promotion of calcium absorption and reduction of bone breakdown.

In men, bone density can be compromised (given the effect on estrogen production), as can overall lean muscle mass, strength, size, and energy secondary to a reduction in circulating levels of testosterone. Beyond this, consuming a diet severely low or absent in fat can not only lead to symptoms of deficiency, but can also result in organ failure and even death.

Saturated fats are solid at room temperature and found mostly in animal foods, such as milk, cheese, and meat, although they can also be present in tropical oils like coconut oil, palm oil, and cocoa butter. Most experts suggest limiting your intake of these types of fats because of their potential for raising your LDL (bad) cholesterol.

That being said, newer research is showing that saturated fats may actually not be as bad for you as we once thought. You may still want to cautiously consume saturated fats, but you don't necessarily need to fear them, as we once did.

One example of a saturated fat that actually has health benefits is coconut oil, which is also referred to as a medium-chain triglyceride (MCT). Although most nutritionists warn against going overboard on your consumption of this tasty oil, in small amounts it may actually be good for you.

When it comes to the trans-saturated fatty acids ("trans fats"), avoid these at all costs. These compounds are used to harden fat and increase shelf life, and are commonly found in processed foods, crackers, piecrusts, cookies, some types of margarine, and some salad dressings. This type of fat is extremely unhealthy and not what your body needs for good health.

An Expert Opinion by **William S. Harris**, **PhD** in the March 19, 2007 *American Journal of Cardiology* (Vol. 99 - 6A) retrospectively evaluated the effects of omega-3 fatty acids on patients undergoing coronary artery bypass grafting (n=2), carotid endarterectomy (n=2), and femoral artery catheterization (n=15). On review of these studies, he stated, "In these studies, the risk for clinically significant bleeding was virtually non-existent."

He went on to point to another previous study, "Dietary fatty acids in human thrombosis and hemostasis" (Knapp HR. *Am J Clin Nutr* 1997: 65(suppl): 1687S-1698S), which also found no link between administration of omega-3 fatty acids and increased bleeding in cardiovascular studies. He added that this study further found no correlation between administrations of omega-3 fatty acids and increased bleeding in pregnant women during delivery or in dialysis patients.

He concluded that "…the experience has been virtually unanimous: omega-3 fatty acid supplements do not increase the risk for clinically significant bleeding, even in patients being treated with anti-platelet or anti-thrombotic medications."

According to these reviews, fish oils may actually contribute far less to thinning of our blood and clotting problems than previously suspected. If so, their anti-inflammatory properties may actually be a benefit around the time of surgery. Again, please check with your surgeon and get his or her approval before surgery.

Carbohydrates

Our next macronutrient is the carbohydrate. While this too has been maligned in recent years, it is an essential component that is necessary for maintaining normal bodily functions. Carbohydrates are comprised of various sugar molecules and are critical for fueling the body. Of the sugars, the most critical one is glucose, which is the primary fuel used by the brain. When burned, it releases a total of four kilocalories of energy per gram. To help provide a constant source of energy for the body, glucose is stored in the liver as glycogen and broken down as needed for additional fuel.

All carbohydrates are broken down for energy, but release sugar at different rates, depending upon their molecular structure and the presence of fiber. This is why you're better off eating an apple than drinking apple juice. Natural fiber within the apple itself helps slow the release of sugar into your bloodstream and ultimately can help temper the triggered release of insulin that occurs when drinking apple juice alone.

To help determine how fast a specific food is broken down and the sugar released into your bloodstream, we talk about the glycemic index.

The higher the number, the faster your blood sugar will rise and the more effect a specific food will have on the speed and the volume of insulin release. However, other factors can also affect a food's glycemic index, including how long you cook it, how ripe the food is, and what other foods you are eating in addition to it. Many nutritionists suggest combining a protein with a carbohydrate to help temper and slow down the release of its sugar.

The glycemic index is not the only thing to consider when choosing healthy food. Look for essential vitamins and minerals in the food you eat, as well.

If a food has a low index but is devoid of any nutritional value, then the index number doesn't really matter, does it?

To better understand the actual effects of specific carbohydrates on our blood-sugar levels, nutritionists point to an even more important number: the glycemic load. The glycemic load of a serving of food can be calculated as its carbohydrate content measured in grams (g), multiplied by the food's GI, and divided by 100.

GL = GI/100 x Net Carbohydrates

(Net carbohydrates are equal to the total carbohydrates minus dietary fiber)

This number is potentially more helpful than the glycemic index alone because it takes into account the actual amount of carbohydrates in a specific food and not just how easily it is broken down to glucose. This additional information tells you how likely it is to raise your blood sugar and to what extent. As a rule of thumb, glycemic loads below 10 are considered by most nutritional experts to be low, while glycemic loads above 20 are considered to be high. Considering that glycemic load is related to the food's effect on blood sugar, low glycemic load meals are commonly recommended for diabetic control, as well as weight loss.

For most health challenges (especially diabetes and hypoglycemia), fat burning, minimizing inflammation, tissue healing, heart and brain health, and for optimization of overall health, we recommend that you consume whole-food carbohydrates predominantly in the number-one BEST (low glycemic) category, only occasionally in the number-two OK (medium glycemic) category, and always with an emphasis on organic sourcing.

BEST (low glycemic carbohydrates):

These are low on the glycemic index (a rating of approximately 10 to 40). Eat these carbs *most often* throughout the day and *as much as possible* with quality protein, some "good" fat, and fiber.

☐ Acidic fruits: Grapefruit and lemon juice (i.e., added to drinks and foods)
☐ Berries: Acai, blueberries, cranberries, raspberries, and strawberries
☐ Cruciferous vegetables: Broccoli, green or red cabbage, and cauliflower
☐ Dry root vegetables: Jerusalem artichoke, kohlrabi, and turnip
☐ Green, leafy vegetables: Bok choy, lettuce (green, red, romaine, and mixed greens), kale, and parsley
☐ Green stalk vegetables: Artichoke, asparagus, green beans, and fresh green peas (in the pod)
☐ Legumes: Dried beans like adzuki, black, navy, etc. (preferably soaked overnight first for much better digestion and/or sprouted or fermented), tiger nuts (new, top choice), lentils, dried peas, and black-eyed peas
☐ Natural sweeteners: Stevia herb (green or white), Lo Han, birch tree extract (Xylitol; consume in moderation because it may cause flatulence at intake levels greater than approximately four grams/serving), fructose (only in moderation and that which is found naturally occurring in certain whole fruits; not the form found in concentrated fructose powder or high fructose corn syrup)
☐ Orange and yellow vegetables: All winter squash varieties and all summer squash varieties
☐ Sub-acid fruits: Apples (more sour, less sweet varieties; e.g., Granny Smith and some apples that are just ripe but not overripe), kiwis, plums, and tomatoes
☐ Watery vegetables: Cucumbers, celery, daikon radish, fennel bulb, and red radish

- ☐ Whole (slow-cooking) grains (soaked overnight first, then cooked slowly and not overcooked): Whole grain, buckwheat, quinoa, and 100% (black) wild rice
- ☐ Acidic fruits: Lemons Berries: Blueberries
- ☐ Cruciferous vegetables: Broccoli and red cabbage
- ☐ Dry root vegetables: Kohlrabi and rutabaga
- ☐ Green, leafy vegetables (juiced raw or lightly steamed): Kale
- ☐ Green and/or watery vegetable juices (fresh-squeezed and single or in combination): Wheatgrass, kale, bok choy, celery, cucumber, daikon, fennel bulb, and parsley
- ☐ Green stalk vegetables: Artichoke and asparagus
- ☐ Orange and yellow fruits and vegetables: All winter squash varieties
- ☐ Sub-acidic fruits: Granny Smith apples, plums, tomatoes

OKAY (medium glycemic carbohydrates):

These are in the middle of the glycemic index (rating at approximately 40 to 65); consume them in *moderation* and *always* with quality protein, some good fat, and fiber.

- ☐ Fresh fruit and green or watery vegetable juices combined with apple, lemon, plum, wheatgrass, kale, bok choy, celery, cucumber, daikon, fennel, and parsley (You may consume about 10 to 15 minutes before a meal, with a meal, or in a protein shake.)
- ☐ Breads (high-fiber, whole-grain): Ezekiel 4:9 sprouted
- ☐ Legumes: Dried peas—green, split yellow, and green
- ☐ Sub-acidic fruits: Apples, cherries, fresh figs, pears, peaches
- ☐ Starchy vegetables (non-GMO, organic): Corn(frozen, on the cob), green peas (fresh/frozen), sweet potatoes, and yams
- ☐ Sweeteners: Coconut nectar crystals W
- ☐ Whole grains : Whole-grain brown rice (basmati, medium- and long-grain, and Wehani); whole-grain millet; whole or semi-whole-grain oats (only if no gluten sensitivity or allergy; this is the best choice for medium glycemic grains)

SOMETIMES OKAY (high glycemic but nutrient-dense carbohydrates):

These rate at approximately 65 to 100+, but they are high in micronutrients. Consume them only if you are exercising regularly for muscle mass, following surgery, or participating in high-endurance athletic training and competition.

These foods should ideally be consumed with your post-exercise protein shake or as a meal to replenish used glycogen energy (normally stored in the skeletal muscles and the liver). Replenishing this glycogen (stored glucose in the body) is critical for gaining muscle mass or while recovering from high-endurance training and competition (e.g., long-distance running). Consume these foods only if you are not diabetic, not hypoglycemic, not on an anti-candida diet, and/or not trying to burn excess body fat. *Always* consume them with quality protein, some good fat, and fiber.

- ☐ Chips (100% whole-grain-based): Corn (organic, non-GMO, sprouted or un-sprouted, no oil added, not fried, unsalted, and baked), brown rice (whole-grain, ideally sprouted, no oil added, not fried, and baked)
- ☐ Dried fruits: Dried figs, prunes, and raisins
- ☐ Melons: Cantaloupe, honeydew, watermelon
- ☐ Grains (organic, non-GMO): Instant oatmeal, steel-cut oats
- ☐ Sprouted "dessert-like" cake/bread (organic, non-GMO): Manna® brand (Essene, organic, very high-fiber, sprouted)
- ☐ Sweet fruits: Bananas (not overripe), dates, grapes, mangos, papaya, and pineapple
- ☐ Sweeteners (organic, non-GMO): Sweet fruits (above), organic and raw (unheated) honey, cane juice or juice powder (evaporated/unrefined, high mineral content)
- ☐ Vegetables: Carrots (raw, lightly steamed, or mixed in fresh green juices)

- ☐ (Whole-grain baked, organic, non-GMO) Cereals: These are mostly found with cereals in the health-food section of the store. There are no added processed sugars, they're made from/with 100% whole grains and healthy oils, and they're sweetened with only less-damaging, more whole-food-form sugars, like dried fruits, evaporated cane juice, raw honey, or stevia (whole-food green or white), etc. They use brown rice; buckwheat; quinoa; millet; teff; and barley, oats, wheat, rye (if you are not gluten-intolerant). Examples are oat flakes, rice flakes, granola, muesli, wheat flakes, etc.(Whole-grain, organic, non-GMO)
- ☐ Flour products: These are made with 100% whole grains, healthy oils, and sweeteners (see above). They use brown rice; buckwheat; quinoa; millet; teff; and barley, oat, wheat, and rye (if you're not gluten-intolerant). Examples of foods are breads, muffins, pancakes, pasta, waffles, etc.

BAD (high glycemic carbohydrates): These are very high on the glycemic index; they rate at approximately 71 to 100 or greater. They have very little or no nutritional content and/or have some negative food components. For instance, potatoes are a nightshade vegetable that contain a potentially joint-irritating substance called solanic acid. ***Try to avoid this list of foods all of the time!***

- ☐ All-white refined flour and grains (usually sourced from refined wheat but can also be processed from barley, oats, rice or other grains): Breads, muffins, pancakes, pasta, waffles, white rice cakes, instant and/or quick-cooking white rice, etc.
- ☐ Fruit juices: Processed, glassed, or in cartons; pasteurized and unrefrigerated juices. Instead, eat whole fruit, or drink fresh-squeezed juices.
- ☐ Refined cereals (with/without sugar added): Corn flakes, puffed rice, Kellogg's (all kinds), General Mills (all kinds), and most other mainstream cereal companies that contain GMOs

- ☐ Refined corn flour foods: Tortillas, taco shells, chips, etc
- ☐ Sweeteners: Refined sugars, like glucose (isolated and concentrated), white sugar, brown sugar, corn syrup, high fructose corn syrup, turbinado sugar
- ☐ Vegetables: White potatoes

PROTEINS

Protein is the third major macronutrient and a component of every cell in your body. It is critical for growth and repair and often referred to as the "building block of life". In addition, it is necessary for the production of hormones, enzymes, and other essential body chemicals. Unlike carbohydrates and fat, protein cannot actually be stored, so we require a constant supply from our diets. As an energy source, it is the last macronutrient to be burned for energy. When utilized, it releases a total of four kilocalories of energy per gram.

Each molecule of protein is comprised of individual amino acids designated as essential, non-essential, or conditional. Essential amino acids cannot be made by the body and must be ingested via our diets (histidine, isoleucine, leucine, lysine, methionine, phenylalanine, threonine, tryptophan, and valine). Non-essential amino acids are actually produced by our bodies and do not need to be ingested (alanine, asparagine, aspartic acid, glutamic acid). Conditional amino acids are generally not essential but may become so under times of severe stress or illness (arginine, cysteine, glutamine, tyrosine, glycine, ornithine, proline, and serine). Our dependence on them within our diets really depends on what is going on at the time.

Common forms of protein include fish, poultry, red meat, beans, and nuts. Supplemental protein can also be added to your diet in the form of whey protein, egg protein, soy protein, and various forms of vegan protein (e.g., brown rice, pea, hemp, and others).
While these protein sources can all boost your overall intake, they have individual advantages and disadvantages that may make you favor one form over the other.

The use of supplementary forms of protein has become more common over the last decade, but it's often challenging to know which specific form is best suited to your goals.

The following is a list of the major supplemental proteins, along with their inherent advantages and disadvantages. Based on this information, you can decide which one is best for you:

Currently Available Forms of Supplemental Protein

1. Rice
   a. Advantages:
      i. Low cost
      ii. Hypoallergenic
   b. Disadvantages
      i. Almost always contains low levels of mercury, lead, and/or tungsten
      ii. Incomplete protein so needs to be added to pumpkin seed, or another complimentary protein source
2. Pea
   a. Advantages:
      i. Low cost
      ii. Hypoallergenic
   b. Disadvantages:
      i. Pricey
      ii. Incomplete protein so needs to be added to rice, pumpkin seed, or another complimentary protein source
3. Sacha inchi
   a. Advantages:
      i. Multi-nutrient dense
      ii. Hypoallergenic

   b. Disadvantages:
      i. Pricey
      ii. Incomplete protein so needs to be added to rice, pumpkin seed,or another complimentary protein source

4. Pumpkin seed
    a. Advantages:
        i. Multi-nutrient dense
        ii. Hypoallergenic
        iii. Anti-microbial
    b. Disadvantages:
        i. Incomplete protein so needs to be added to rice, pumpkin seed, or another complimentary protein source
5. Whey
    a. Advantages:
        i. Most balanced and complete amino acid profile
    b. Disadvantages:
        i. Potentially allergenic
6. Collagen peptides (low molecular weight)
    a. Advantages:
        i. Very balanced and complete amino acid profile
        ii. Ideal for pre and post-operative protein/micro-nutritional support and healing
    b. Disadvantages:
        i. Moderately pricey
7. Egg whites
    a. Advantages:
        i. Second most balanced and complete amino acid profile
    b. Disadvantages:
        i. Potentially allergenic
8. Cricket protein
    a. Advantages:
        i. Very complete amino acid profile
        ii. Moderately dense in protein
        iii. High in vitamin B12
        iv. Ecologically sustainable

b. Disadvantages:
- i. Possibly slow cultural acceptance of consuming insects as a food source; Moderately expensive {for now)

9. Hemp
    a. Advantages:
    - i. Compliments other vegetarian proteins (e.g., pea, rice,
    - ii. Ecologically sustainable
    b. Disadvantages:
    - i. Incomplete protein (alone)
    - ii. Moderate food sensitivities in some individuals

FIBER

Fiber is the next macronutrient, and comes in both soluble and insoluble forms. The soluble form dissolves in water and can slow digestion, while the insoluble form is obviously not soluble and has no effect on the rate of absorption of other food in the gut. This last form is important as a prebiotic food source for bacteria within your gut and may potentially improve overall gut health. Regardless of the type of fiber, neither form is burned for energy nor has any caloric value.

Various supplemental forms of fiber are available if you are not consuming enough fruits and vegetables in your diet or if current demands require you to increase your protein intake. I recommend that patients increase both their soluble and insoluble fiber intake after surgery for several reasons.

First, most experience constipation after surgery as a result of hormonal shifts, as well as the slew of medications that are prescribed. In this case, soluble fiber can help produce a good bowel movement per day and help keep you regular.

Next, because we generally use antibiotics both during and after surgery, there is a good chance that we are wiping out not only the bad bacteria but also the very important bacteria in your gut. To help replenish good bacteria and encourage your intestinal tract to repopulate efficiently with good bacteria, we ask patients to consume a probiotic with an insoluble fiber prebiotic to help re-establish the bacterial flora within their guts.

On a side note, several studies have revealed a direct correlation between the presence of "good" bacteria in the gut, overall gut health, and the prevention of several disease processes. To emphasize the importance of your intestinal tract, keep in mind that as much as 70% of your immune cells reside there and that up to 60% of the neurotransmitters that help run your central nervous system are produced there.

Although antibiotics may be a necessary evil, the temporary damage they may cause to our gut occurs in a time when you depend on the health of your gut more than ever. Once again, this underscores not only the importance of a source of good bacteria (probiotics) but also of a critical food source to nourish them (prebiotics).

On that note, the term "prebiotics" refers to specific types of dietary fiber that effectively encourage an increase or proliferation of beneficial intestinal bacteria (or "probiotics"). While you can ingest prebiotics, your body actually cannot digest them; however, your body's bacteria can and will use them as a source of food. Prebiotics consist of soluble fibers that are most commonly either inulin or fructooligosaccharides (FOS), which can be naturally found in certain foods or ingested as isolated supplements.

While this unique type of soluble fiber nourishes primarily the Bifido strains of bacteria that reside predominantly in your lower intestinal tract or colon, to some extent they also act as food for the Lactobacilli bacteria that prefer the upper intestinal tract or small bowel.

In the last several years, more and more studies are confirming the positive health effects of beneficial gut bacteria. Some of the ways in which beneficial gut bacterial can potentially improve your health include the following:

- Improved regularity of bowel movements – You should be having at least one bowel movement/day for optimal health.
- Improved immunity – Keep in mind that up to 70% of your immune cells actually reside within your gut!
- Repair of leaky gut syndrome – This is known to be triggered by stress or trauma to the body. Some practitioners think that the trauma of surgery itself may be a strong trigger for development of post-operative leaky gut syndrome.

☐ Increased bio-availability of absorption of dietary calcium – This is very important not only for daily bodily functions but also for the maintenance of bone homeostasis.

Prebiotics can be found in a number of healthy foods but are most concentrated in the following:

1. Raw chicory root: 64.6% prebiotic fiber by weight
2. Raw Jerusalem artichoke: 31.5% prebiotics by weight
3. Raw dandelion greens: 24.3% prebiotic fiber by weight
4. Raw garlic: 17.5% prebiotics by weight
5. Raw leek: 11.7% prebiotic fiber by weight
6. Raw onion: 8.6% prebiotics by weight
7. Cooked onion: 5% prebiotic fiber by weight
8. Raw asparagus: 5% prebiotics by weight
9. Raw wheat bran: 5% prebiotic fiber by weight
10. Wheat flour, baked: 4.8% prebiotics by weight
11. Raw banana: 1% prebiotic fiber by weight

(Courtesy of *www.prebiotin.com*)

These values refer only to foods in their raw forms (unless indicated). Cooking may significantly alter their prebiotic content.

To help bolster the beneficial bacteria within your gut, you can either take a prebiotic supplement, or you can try some of the following foods:
- Miso
- Coconut water kefir
- Dairy-free yogurts
- Kombucha
- Kimchi
- Sauerkraut
- Tempeh
- Raw cacao

WATER

The final macronutrient is water and really needs no introduction. As you may guess, water is critical to our health because it hydrates and properly detoxifies. Depending upon the amount and the type of food you are ingesting, as well as your overall hydration status, your body requires a certain amount of water each and every day.

The amount of water recommended for you after surgery depends upon several factors, including not only your baseline medical health but also the procedure being performed. Check with your surgeon to see what they recommend for you.

Unless you are unable to take food by mouth or have pre-existing kidney disease, you should be fine consuming a minimum of 8 to 12 glasses of water per day. I recommend slightly more for my patients, since we live in a very dry part of the country, where we experience higher than normal evaporative losses. However much you plan to consume, remember that you are also taking in water from specific foods that you eat, so a glass here and there can potentially be accounted for by some of the food that you consume.

A good measure of your overall hydration is the character of your urine. If your urine is slightly colored to clear, you are probably well hydrated. Bright yellow urine may mean that you are dehydrated or that you recently took a multi-vitamin. Foul-smelling dark urine is something you definitely don't want and suggests that you are very dry and need to rehydrate. Don't ever let yourself get to that stage. Hydration is not that hard if you simply keep up with it.

I encourage my patients to add lemon wedges or a small amount of fresh lemon juice to their water to shift their body to a more alkaline pH balance. Many foods are acidifying and push the pH balance of our bodies to a state where our enzymatic reactions function less efficiently.

This is made even worse during periods of high protein consumption, which in itself has a known tendency to push our body's pH balance to the acidic side. A simple remedy for this is to squeeze half a lemon into a glass of water first thing in the morning. Consume the water, and then rinse your mouth to avoid etching of your teeth from the acetic acid. This simple trick may mean all the difference in helping your body maintain itself in a more efficient alkaline state.

Micronutrients

"The human body heals itself and nutrition provides the resources to accomplish the task."
- **Roger Williams**, **PhD** (Pioneer in biochemistry, nutrition, biochemical individuality, and public education)

Micronutrients include vitamins, minerals, and herbs. While these are required in much smaller amounts than the macronutrients, they are still critical for optimal health and may become more necessary during times of increased stress or illness.

VITAMINS: Water-Soluble vs. Fat-Soluble

Broadly speaking, vitamins can be broken down into those that are fat-soluble (stored in our fat) and those that are water-soluble (dissolved in water). The major difference here is that because fat-soluble vitamins can be stored in fat, they can build up toxic levels if you ingest levels that are too high. The body uses what it needs at the time and stores the rest in fat cells for future use.

This is not the case with water-soluble vitamins. The body shuttles these vitamins into the bloodstream, uses what it needs, and excretes the remainder into the urine. An exception to the process of fat-soluble vitamin storage occurs in patients with cystic fibrosis, who do not store or process fats normally. These patients actually do require more frequent ingestion of the fat-soluble vitamins since they are unable to store them. Keep in mind that too much of a good thing (even a water-soluble vitamin) can be a bad thing. Researchers are finding that even water-soluble vitamins can potentially be toxic if taken at very high levels. Check with your doctor before undertaking mega-dosing, even though it may seem like a good thing.

Storage is not the only problem. For some vitamins, you also need other nutrients to guarantee proper absorption. A good example of this is the relationship between Magnesium levels and absorption of Vitamins A and D. Without the proper amount of circulating magnesium, these fat-soluble vitamins are simply not absorbed.

Let's begin by talking about the fat-soluble vitamins, which include the following:

☐ **Pro-Vitamin A/Vitamin A**

- o Sources:
    - Spinach, broccoli, milk, eggs, liver, and fish
- o Functions:
    - Plays an essential role in vision, reproduction, cellular growth, and healthy immune function
- o Warnings:
    - Because these vitamins are stored in fat, high doses may ultimately lead to toxic levels and cause brain damage, etc.
    - Low magnesium levels may hamper proper absorption.
- o Recommended adult average daily dose range: 5,000 - 10,000 IUs

☐ **Vitamin D3**

- o Sources:
    - Fatty fish, eggs, organ meats, milk, and sunlight

o Functions:
  - Thought to be more of a pro-hormone than an actual vitamin
  - Critical for maintaining proper blood levels of calcium by increasing calcium absorption from food and limiting calcium loss through urine
  - May help facilitate the transfer of calcium from bone to bloodstream
  - Along with vitamin K2 and a few other key micronutrients, important for maintaining healthy bones and teeth
  - Deficiencies can impact the optimal function of:
    - Immune system
    - Skin
    - Heart
    - Muscles
    - Brain

o Warnings:
  - This is a fat-soluble nutrient, so excess levels may build up in the body, though new research and higher recommended intake levels suggests it is less likely to occur.
  - Low magnesium levels may hamper proper absorption.

o Recommended adult average daily dose range: 1,000 - 4,000 IUs

- **Vitamin E (Intake should ideally include a balance of all or most sub-fractions, including alpha/beta/gamma-tocopherols/tocotrienols.)**
  - o Sources:
    - Nuts and seeds, avocado, vegetables and vegetable oils, whole grains, organ meats, and eggs
  - o Functions:
    - Protection of cell membranes and other fat-soluble constituents of the body (e.g., LDL cholesterol)
    - May help reduce the risk of heart attacks
    - May play a role in the body's ability to process glucose, so may be helpful in prevention/treatment of diabetes
    - May directly affect inflammation, blood-cell regulation, connective tissue growth, and the genetic control of cellular division
  - o Warnings:
    - Low chance of toxicity levels; however, due to the fact that these vitamins are stored in fat, high doses may possibly lead to toxic levels and symptoms such as nausea; diarrhea; stomach cramps; headache; blurred vision; rash; fatigue; weakness; and may cause hyper vitaminosis E, which may increase bleeding and bruising problems and potentially lead to a Vitamin K deficiency.
    - o Recommended adult average daily dose range: Controversial but safely 30 IUs (if alpha alone) - 400 IUs (if mixed carotenoids)

☐ **Vitamin K**
  o Sources:
    ▪ Green, leafy vegetables; natto (fermented soy product); supplement (ideally a combination of K1 and K2)
  o Functions:
    ▪ Comes in three forms: K1, K2 (recommended form), and K3
    ▪ K1: Proper blood clotting; K2: shuttling serum calcium <u>away</u> from soft tissues (i.e., arteries) and into the bone matrix
  o Warnings:
    ▪ If you are on blood-thinning medications (i.e., COUMADIN®) or have any blood coagulation disorders, check with your health practitioner before consuming a Vitamin K1/K2 supplement and/or consuming high Vitamin K foods.
  o Recommended adult average daily dose range: 70 - 100 mcg (Vitamin K2)

Water-soluble vitamins include the following:

☐ **Vitamin B1 (Thiamine)**
  o Sources:
    ▪ Whole grains, meat, nuts, yeast products, and legumes
  o Functions:
    ▪ Required for the breakdown of carbohydrates, fats, and proteins
    ▪ Essential component in the production of ATP (adenosine tri-phosphate) for energy

- Critical to the proper functioning of nerve cells
- Warnings:
  - ☐ Low level of oral toxicity
  o Recommended adult average daily dose range: 1.5 mg to 8 mg

☐ **Vitamin B2 (Riboflavin)**

  o Sources:
  - Leafy-green vegetables, fish, eggs, dairy, meat and organ meats, and whole grains
  o Functions:
  - Important for the processing of amino acids and fats
  - Important for the activation of Vitamins B6/B9
  - Important component in the conversion of carbohydrates to ATP for energy
  - May act as an antioxidant under certain conditions
  - Warnings:
    - ☐ Low toxicity levels
    - ☐ Higher intake levels may harmlessly turn urine a brighter yellow color.
  o Recommended adult average daily dose range: 1.67 - 4 mg

☐ **Vitamin B3 (Niacin)**

  o Sources:
  - Poultry, meats, nuts, whole grains, fish, and dairy products
  o Functions:

- Required for cellular respiration
- Critical component in the release of energy from carbohydrates, fats, and proteins
- Important for the support of proper circulation, healthy skin, optimal functioning of the nervous system, and normal secretion of bile/stomach acids
- May be effective in the treatment of schizophrenia and other mental illnesses
- May enhance memory

o Warnings:
- May cause skin flushing
- Be careful using high doses for cholesterol-lowering and good HDL-increasing therapy. May increase the potential for liver damage

o Recommended adult average daily dose range: 20 mg. to 45 mg.

□ **Vitamin B5 (Pantothenic Acid)**

o Sources:
- Peas, beans, whole grains, meats, poultry, and fruits

o Functions:
- Plays an important role in the metabolism of and release of energy from sugar and fats
- Important factor in the production of fats
- Plays a role in modifying the shape of proteins

o Warnings:
- Low-level toxicity

o Recommended adult average daily dose range: 10 mg. to 45 mg.

☐ **Vitamin B6 (Pyridoxine)**

    o Sources:

- Bananas, beans, potatoes, meats and organ meats, fish, poultry, legumes, nuts, and leafy-green vegetables

    o Functions:

- Important component in the synthesis of antibodies by the immune system
- Helps to maintain nervous system function
- Aids in the formation of red blood cells
- Critical component in chemical reactions necessary for digestion of proteins; the higher your protein intake, the more you require Vitamin B6.

    o Warnings:

- With too high an intake, neurological disorders can potentially occur.

    o Recommended adult average daily dose range: 2 mg. to 10 mg.

☐ **Vitamin B9 (Folic Acid)**

    o Sources:

- Eggs; dairy; asparagus; orange juice; dark, leafy-green vegetables; beans; brown bread; and tea

    o Functions:

- Folate is naturally occurring in food; folic acid is the synthetic form

- Important in the metabolism of amino acids and the production of proteins, nucleic acids, and blood cells
- Although folic acid has been shown to reduce homocysteine levels, its ability to reduce heart disease has been called into question in recent studies

o Warnings:

- In normal doses, folate is very safe, but if given in mega-doses (usually above 15,000 mcg), you may experience stomach problems, sleep disturbance, skin reactions, and seizures.
- While it has been suggested to be preventative of various cancers, recent studies have suggested that it may actually increase progression of these cancers when they are already present. If you have a history of colon cancer or polyps, you may want to lower your intake of folic acid, since it could potentiate the growth of cancer by reducing the effectiveness of your body's own, cancer-fighting "natural killer cells".

o Recommended adult average daily dose:

- 400 mcg/day
- Isolated supplement form should ideally be taken on an empty stomach, since food may delay or reduce overall absorption
- Higher doses may mask an underlying B12 deficiency.

- **Vitamin B12 (Methyl-Cobalamin [Superior Form] or Cyanocobalamin)**
  - o Sources:
    - Dairy products, eggs, fish, meats, and fermented foods
  - o Functions:
    - Critical for nervous system function and replication of DNA
    - The active methyl component is utilized in the production of S-adenosylmethionine or SAMe, which may be effective in the treatment of osteoarthritis, as well as various mental disorders like depression.
    - Participates with folic acid to reduce homocysteine levels
  - o Warnings:
    - If you have Leber's hereditary optic neuropathy (affecting your eyes), caution should be taken when consuming supplemental Vitamin B12. Avoid taking supplemental forms if allergic to cobalt or cobalamin.
  - o Recommended adult average daily dose range: 50 - 100 mcg
    - Sublingual (dissolved underneath the tongue) methyl-cobalamin is most efficient for increased absorption, especially as you age and lose intrinsic factor production and therefore have lowered GI absorption. Sublingual B12 can also help to positively support mental and physical relaxation and sleep quality.

□ **Vitamin H (Biotin)**

o Sources:

- Dairy products, meat and poultry, oats and grains, soybeans and legumes, mushrooms, and nuts

o Functions:

- Actually considered to be a member of the Vitamin B family
- Actively involved in energy production, as well as synthesis of fatty acids
- Supports optimal nervous system function, as well as potentially promoting healthy hair, skin, and nails

o Warnings:

- High intake dose problems are very rare.

o Recommended adult average daily dose: 300 mcg

□ **Vitamin C**

o Sources:

- Berries, fruits (especially citrus), red peppers, tomatoes, broccoli, spinach, and sprouts
- Camu camu berries are an excellent source!

o Functions:

- Potent antioxidant
- Protects LDL cholesterol (bad cholesterol) from oxidative damage
- Key component in collagen production
- Critical for optimal wound healing
- Aids in the formation of liver bile

o Warnings:

- High doses may cause gastrointestinal distress and diarrhea. Test for maximum dosage tolerability by implementing the Bowel Tolerance Test.

o Recommended adult average daily dose range: 60 mg (Daily value) - 2,000 mg+ (For some chronic illnesses, it can slow the progression of hardening of the arteries; for acute illnesses like colds, sore throats, etc.)

MINERALS

Minerals are critical to a wide range of bodily functions and are broken down into macro minerals (minerals our bodies need in larger amounts) and trace minerals (which our bodies require in far smaller amounts). Examples of macro minerals include calcium, phosphorus, magnesium, sodium, potassium, chloride, and sulfur. Examples of trace minerals include iron, manganese, copper, iodine, zinc, cobalt, fluoride, and selenium.

☐ **Calcium**
  o Sources:
    ▪ Dairy products, fish with bones, whole grains, seeds and nuts, green vegetables, and beans
  o Functions:
    ▪ Aids in bone formation
    ▪ Required for proper blood clotting, signal transmission in nerve cells, and muscle contraction
    ▪ May play a role in lowering blood pressure
  o Warnings:
    ▪ Calcium taken in excessive amounts can potentially cause soft tissue and vascular calcification, renal insufficiency, hypercalcemia, and kidney stones. To minimize these, balance appropriately your intake of calcium with appropriate amounts of magnesium, D3, K2, boron, etc.
  o Recommended adult average daily dose range: 800 - 1,200 mg (depending on dietary intake, age, gender, bone health, etc.)

Chlorine

- o What:
  - Mineral (present in the body as the chloride ion)
- o Sources:
  - Table salt, tap/bottled water, celery, tomatoes, seafood, pickled foods, and salted foods
- o Functions:
  - Essential to life
  - Responsible in part for the maintenance of membrane potential in nerves, nutrient absorption, and transport
  - Helps maintain proper balance of blood volume and pressure
- o Warnings:
  - Excessive amounts of chlorine in (sodium) chloride form may increase or exacerbate blood pressure in certain individuals.
- o Recommended adult average daily dose range: 1,800 - 2,300 mg

Chromium

- o Sources:
  - Fermented foods, whole grains, dairy products, meats, grapes and raisins, beets, and black pepper
- o Functions:
  - Essential in production of glucose tolerance factor (GTF)

- GTF is responsible for potentiating the effect of insulin, and may actually help to lower blood-sugar levels, although results are inconclusive at this point.
- It also may improve glucose transport into fat cells and muscle cells of the heart (cardiomyocytes).
- Active component in the synthesis of fatty acids and cholesterol

  o Warnings:
- The polynicotinate form (as opposed to the picolinate form) in <u>some</u> studies may be safer and more absorbable.
- If diabetic and using medications to control blood sugars, consult with your healthcare practitioner before adding this supplement to your daily regimen.

  o Recommended adult average daily dose range: 90 - 120 mcg

☐ **Copper**

  o Sources:
- Seafood, whole grains and nuts, meats and organ meats, legumes and green vegetables, and molasses

  o Functions:
- Necessary for proper absorption and utilization of iron

  o Critical component in a number of varied chemical reactions throughout your body, including the formation of red blood cells, enzymatic-based antioxidant activity, and energy cycles

- o Warnings:
  - Some individuals are sensitive to even small amounts of supplemental copper intake, with short-term symptoms of nausea, vomiting, and diarrhea. However, copper toxicity is rare. For general health support and proper absorption, consume in an approximate nutrient balance of 1:15 with zinc. Therefore, if taking 1 mg of copper, also consume approximately 15 mg of zinc.
- o Recommended adult average daily dose range: 750 mcg. to 2 mg.
  - Necessary in trace amounts

- ☐ **Magnesium**
  - o Sources:
    - Meat, dairy products, fish, whole grains, green vegetables, nuts and beans, and fruits
  - o Functions:
    - Necessary for the optimal formation of protein, bone, and fatty acids
    - Key component in cellular growth
    - Functions in the activation of B vitamins
    - Participates in over 300 enzymatic reactions in the body, including the processes of muscle relaxation and clotting your blood, and the formation of ATP for energy
    - May potentially lower blood pressure

o Warnings: Magnesium blood toxicity (hypermagnesemia) is very rare and usually only occurs in certain chronically ill patients.
(In fact, the latest nutritional information on magnesium is that most individuals are actually very <u>deficient</u> in this crucial mineral and could potentially increase their overall health and well-being by adding a magnesium supplement and/or increasing magnesium-rich foods in their diets.)

o Recommended adult average daily dose range: The new recommendation is closer to a 1:1 ratio with high-quality calcium or approximately 800 - 1,000 mg. (The old recommendation was closer to a 1:2 ratio with calcium or approximately 400 mg.)

☐ **Manganese**

o Sources:
- Seeds and nuts, whole grains, leafy green vegetables, berries and fruit, eggs, avocado, tea, and seaweed

o Functions:
- Required in small amounts for the manufacture of enzymes necessary in the metabolism of proteins and fat
- Supports optimal immune system function, as well as blood-sugar balance
- Participates in the production of cellular energy, reproduction, and bone growth
- Works with Vitamin K to support normal blood clotting

- Warnings:
    - Low risk of toxicity, unless patient has long-term liver disease, iron-deficiency or anemia – these patients should have their dosages monitored closely
- Recommended adult average daily dose range: Adequate intake (AI) levels are 1.8 - 2.6 mg, depending on gender.

- **Molybdenum**
    - What:
        - Trace mineral
    - Sources:
        - Legumes; dark, leafy-green vegetables; whole grains; dairy products; and organ meats
    - Functions:
        - Required for the activity of some enzymes involved in catabolism (including the breakdown of purines/sulfur amino acids)
    - Warnings:
        - Low level of toxicity unless exposed to a large amount of molybdenum in dust and fumes, primarily in mining and metalworking
    - Recommended adult average daily dose: 75 mcg [Daily Value]

- **Phosphorus**
    - What:
        - Macromineral

- Sources:
  - Fermented foods, meats and poultry, whole grains and seeds, dairy and eggs, mushrooms, and vegetables
- Functions:
  - Usually found in nature combined with oxygen as "phosphate"
  - Most phosphate in the body found in your bones
  - Integral part of cell membranes (phospholipids) and lipoprotein molecules
  - Trace amounts participate in biochemical reactions throughout your body
- Warnings:
  - Low level of toxicity
- Recommended adult average daily dose range: 1,000 mg. (1 gram) [Daily Value]

- **Potassium**
  - What:
    - Macromineral
  - Sources:
    - Unprocessed meats; fish; milk; fruits and vegetables, such as leafy greens, bananas, berries, oranges, lemons, avocados, and tomatoes
    - Highly refined food items such as oils, sugar, and fats lack potassium.

o Functions:
- Found in all cells of the body; levels controlled by kidneys
- Essential mineral/electrolyte; helps regulate blood pressure and may reduce risk for cardiovascular disease
- Plays an important role in electrolyte regulation, nerve function, muscle controlWorks with sodium to maintain blood pressure by increasing sodium excretion from the body
- Regulates water and mineral balance throughout the body

o Warnings:
- Excessive potassium intake rarely occurs within healthy individuals with properly functioning kidneys. Excess potassium in the body (hyperkalaemia) may occur in patients with renal disease (compromised kidney function), especially if given too much potassium chloride salt supplementation.
- Cardiovascular and neuromuscular abnormalities can occur with excessive body potassium levels.
- The safest and most natural way to obtain adequate levels of potassium is by consuming the whole foods mentioned above.

o Recommended adult average daily dose range:
- Most Americans do NOT get enough potassium in their diets.

- The adequate intake (AI) daily level range established for adults 18 years and older is 4,700 - 5,100 mg.

☐ **Zinc**

- What:
  - Trace mineral
- Sources:
  - Animal protein, beans, pumpkin seeds
- Functions:
  - Immune support, cell reproduction, tissue growth and repair, wound-healing, used in the body (along with copper) for enzyme-based antioxidant production
- Recommended adult average daily dose range: 10 - 18 mg

HERBS/SPICES/OTHERS

There are a number of ancillary compounds that your body does not necessarily need, but that may improve its functioning and your overall health.

- **Curcumin**
  - o Sources:
    - Found in low levels in the herb turmeric.
    - Because of these low levels, it is best to supplement with curcumin directly instead of turmeric.
  - o Functions:
    - May be combined with black pepper/piperine to increase bioavailability (inhibitor of glucuronidation); can also increase bioavailability by creating nanoparticles, liposomes, micelles, and phospholipid complexes (advantages: longer circulation, increased cellular permeability, induced resistance to metabolic processes)
    - Bromelain increases the anti-inflammatory effect, so it is often combined with curcumin for increased effectiveness.

o Warnings:

- May increase the anti-platelet effect of various medications; check with your surgeon before taking this before or immediately following surgery.

- May increase stomach acid. Clear with your primary physician if you have a history of reflux, stomach ulcers, or other intestinal issues.

o Recommended adult average daily dose range: 200 - 800 mg of ideally Bio-Curcumin®.

☐ **Quercetin**

o What:

- Flavonol antioxidant

o Sources:

- Buckwheat, onions, citrus fruits, berries

o Functions:

- Potent flavonoid
- Reduces swelling and lymphedema
- Blood vessel protection and support
- Allergy reaction support

o Dosage: 500 mg, two times per day

☐ **Ginger**

o What:

- A rhizome

o Functions:

- GI calming effect
- Anti-inflammatory
- May thin blood

- o Dosage: Best to use fresh-cut pieces for optimal enzyme and antioxidant activity or drink as a tea 250 mg - 2 g of powder extract or in encapsulation

- **Bromelain**
  - o What:
    - Dietary enzyme derived from pineapple
  - o Sources:
    - Supplemental form or consumed directly in pineapple
  - o Functions:
    - Reduces swelling and inflammation
  - o Dosage: 90 mg, three times per day

- **Milk Thistle**
  - o What:
    - Herb
  - o Functions:
    - Antioxidant
    - Increases glutathione
    - Liver support
  - o Dosage: 50 - 300 mg standardized, two to three times per day, depending on your health, dietary habits and lifestyle, and/or need to cleanse the liver

- **Holy Basil (Tulsi)**
  - o What:
    - Herb/adaptogen

- Functions:
  - Improves response to stress
  - Potentially modulates cortisol
- Dosage: 100 - 300 mg standardized per day when dealing with extra emotional stress and anxiety

- **Ashwaganda**
  - What:
    - Herb/adaptogen
  - Functions:
    - Improves response to stress
    - Potentially modulates cortisol
    - Potential neuron (brain cell) protector
  - Dosage: 50 - 500 mg, depending on goal

- **L-Thiamine**
  - What:
    - Naturally derived amino acid
  - Sources:
    - Green tea
  - Functions:
    - Antioxidant
    - Increases alpha brain waves, which in turn helps improve focus and has a mind-calming effect
  - Dosage: Supplement of 100 - 200 mg standardized extract per day

- **Cayenne (Capsicum)**
  - What:
    - Spice/pepper

- Functions:
  - May help improve blood-sugar control
  - May support blood vessel circulation
  - May support, in conjunction with other nutrients, a reduction in muscle and joint pain
- Dosage: Standardized 450 mg capsules, one to three times per day, preferably with food; or use in powder/spice form, and add to meals

□ **Cinnamon**
- What:
  - Spice
- Functions:
  - Antibiotic function
  - Antioxidant
  - May help improve blood-sugar control
- Dosage: Standardized 500 - 1,000 mg capsules, one to six times per day, preferably with food; or use in tea and/or add to smoothies or sweet meals

□ **Boswellia:**
- What:
  - Herb
- Functions:
  - 5-LOX enzyme inhibitor reduces systemic inflammation and in particular prostate enlargement or BPA
  - Potentially reduces arthritic and other joint pain

o Dosage: 100 - 250 mg per day of standardized extract with high concentrations of AKBA, taken with first meal of day

☐ **Omega-3 Fatty Acids:**

o What:
  o PUFA (poly-unsaturated fatty acid)
  o Sources/Functions:
    ▪ Comprised of ALA, DHA, and EPA
    ▪ ALA omega-3 (alpha linolenic acid):
    ▪ Vegetable oils, including those from flaxseed, walnuts, and spinach
    ▪ Our bodies cannot make ALA, so we must get it from our diets. However, under the right conditions, our bodies can convert ALA to DHA and EPA. This becomes important in the case of strict vegans, who cannot get DHA or EPA from their diets. The problem with this is that the specific types of foods that we eat may not enable us to effectively convert ALA to DHA/EPA. This issue is rather complex. The easiest option is to simply eat foods high in DHA/EPA or consume supplements that actually contain them.

☐ **DHA omega-3 (docosahexaenoic acid)**

o Sources:
    ▪ Marine oils, including those from cold-water, oily fish; calamari; krill; marine algae; and phytoplankton
    ▪ DHA is naturally found throughout the body but is most abundant in the brain, eyes, and heart.

- o Functions:
  - This critical fatty acid is essential for optimal function and development of cells in the brain, retina, heart, and other parts of the nervous system.
  - As a critical structural component of the brain, DHA makes up approximately 30% of the structural fats in the gray matter of the brain and 97% of the overall omega-3s in the brain.
  - DHA is also a major structural fat in the retina of the eye. As such, it plays an important role in both infant visual development and visual function throughout life.
  - Finally, DHA is a key component of the heart (especially in the conducting tissue) and is important for heart health throughout life.
  - Studies have shown that DHAs play active roles in the following:
    - Infant mental development
    - Optimal brain and nervous system development and function
    - Infant visual function and development of vision
    - Maintenance of normal triglyceride levels, heart rate, and blood pressure
    - Possible role in health of the adult eye

☐ Possible reduction of the risk of cardiovascular disease (Research at this point is inconclusive.)EPA omega-3 (eicosapentaenoic acid)

- Reduction of stiffness and joint pain associated with rheumatoid arthritis; may also boost overall effectiveness of various anti-inflammatory drugs

-

- On their own, they have helped reduce symptoms associated with depression and bipolar disorder, in addition to boosting the effects of various anti-depressant medications.

- Given their ability to lower overall inflammation, they may prove helpful in the treatment of asthma.

- Some recent studies suggest that fish oil may reduce the symptoms of ADHD in children and improve overall mental and cognitive skills.

- Some recent studies suggest that fish oils may help protect against Alzheimer's disease and dementia, in addition to having a positive effect on the progression of memory loss associated with aging.

o Warnings:

- Fish oils are thought to have an anti-platelet effect, so they may increase the risk of bleeding. Most surgeons suggest that you stop taking fish oils at least two weeks prior to surgery. They can be continued only with the guidance of your treating physician.

- Know the source of your omega-3 fatty acids. This pertains more to DHA and EPA, which are generally sourced from cold-water fish, which may contain high levels of mercury and other potential contaminants.

  o Recommended dosages: The FDA has advised that adults may safely consume a total of three grams per day of combined EPA/DHA, with no more than two grams coming from dietary supplements.

- **L-Glutamine**
  o What:
    - Conditionally essential amino acid
  o Sources:
    - Supplemental form or as glutamine peptides in protein powders (especially in whey protein isolates)
  o Functions:
    - Can help rebuild gastrointestinal tract lining
    - Supports skeletal muscle integrity
    - Supports immunity
  o Dosage: 1 - 5 g

- **CoQ10**
  o What:
    - Vitamin-like nutrient naturally produced in the body
  o Sources:
    - Supplemental form, either as ubiquinol or ubiquinone; also naturally occurring in smaller amounts, animal-based proteins

- o Function:
  - Antioxydant
  - Boosts intra-cellular energy
- o Dosage: 50 - 200 mg

- ☐ **Probiotic**
  - o What:
    - Beneficial bacteria (or body flora) that resides primarily in the (upper) small intestine and the (lower) large intestine or colon, as well as other areas of the body
  - o Sources:
    - Supplemental form; fermented food products, such as kombucha, kimchi, and yogurt
  - o Functions:
    - Helps to support bowel regularity
    - Supports immune system
    - Creates proper upper and lower gastrointestinal pH balance
    - To produce certain nutrients, especially some B vitamins
    - o Dosage: Usually 1-100 billion colonizing units per day, depending on goals and/or conditions

- ☐ **Pharma-GABA (Gamma Amino Butyric Acid)**
  - o What:
    - Nonessential amino acid
  - o Sources:
    - Supplemental form; tomatoes

- o Functions:
  - ▪ Calming effect on nervous system
  - ▪ May help support anxiety reduction and sleep
- o Dosage: Approximately 500 - 1000 mg

- ☐ **L-Citrulline**
  - o What:
    - ▪ Amino acid
  - o Sources:
    - ▪ Supplemental form; in rinds of watermelons
  - o Functions:
    - ▪ Alternative amino acid to direct arginine for nitric oxide production in the body, which in turn helps to support healthy blood vessel vasodilation throughout the body
    - ▪ Potential libido support
    - ▪ Potential tissue-healing support
    - ▪ With exercise, potential improvements in energy levels and aerobic and anaerobic exercise endurance
  - o Dosage: 1 - 3 g before exercise or before bed

While this list may appear daunting, these ingredients were actually selected from a much longer list provided toward the end of the book. Could you heal without many of these? Probably. But the simple fact that you have read this far suggests that you are proactive and not interested in leaving your healing to chance.

Medicine Is Finally Catching Up

"A man too busy to take care of his health is like a mechanic too busy to take care of his tools."
- Spanish proverb

Change Is Coming

During the writing of this book, I was shocked by the number of physicians who felt that nutrition was not a big issue, but I was also amazed by the growing number who did. Many physicians expressed interest in this topic and commented that this was something desperately needed for their surgical patients. They even shared stories with me of their efforts.

Over the last several years there has been a growing number of scientific articles released on this topic. It appears that the medical system may slowly be catching on. This is a good sign and a sign that your physician may now be more amenable to change and that you as a proactive consumer may soon be able to choose your surgeon based upon not only their surgical expertise but also their willingness to incorporate nutrition in your surgical plan.

A recent *Wall Street Journal* article focused on a new surgical protocol being investigated at the University of Virginia. This protocol goes against the routine of effectively fasting our patients before surgery and shows promise for not only creating faster recovery for patients but also for reducing the overall need for post-operative narcotics. The article's first paragraph really sets the stage for how this approach is groundbreaking:

"Hospitals are starting to abandon the time-honored drill for surgery patients—including fasting, heavy IV fluids, powerful post-op narcotics and bed rest—amid growing evidence that the lack of nutrients, fluid overload and drug side effects can do more harm than good."

In the study, patients were still told to fast after midnight, but were then given a "...*carbohydrate-loaded drink fortified with electrolytes, minerals, and vitamins*" two to three hours prior to their surgeries and were pre-treated with non-narcotic painkillers and an epidural (which remained after their procedure). Because patients were pre-hydrated, they were able to receive less IV fluid volume during surgery. Researchers found that patients were not only able to ambulate earlier after surgery, and eat solid food, but were also discharged sooner.

Dr. Tracy Hedrick, co-author of the study and Professor of Surgery at UVA, points out:

"This is contradictory to the way we've practiced for 50 years, but it is becoming more and more evident that this really is more effective and better for patients. Surgery is already a significant trauma on the body and we want to help keep patients as normal as possible for as long as possible."

In the study he and his team found that by following this protocol in the colorectal surgery patient population, they were able to reduce the length of hospital stays by 2.2 days and reduce complications by as much as 17%. This led to a whopping $7,129 cost savings per patient!

Dr. Hedrick points out that many physicians and anesthesiologists are reluctant to embrace this new approach and that adoption has been slow. A 2011 study in *JAMA Surgery* found that while clear benefits have been proven from the protocol, many physicians nationally have been reluctant to adapt. In response, the American College of Surgeons has launched a national initiative to help educate surgeons and hopefully increase adoption of this new approach.

Along the same lines, the ERAS (Enhanced Recovery After Surgery) protocols were initially developed by Professor Henrik Kehlet in the 1990s. These surgical fast-track programs have been used in a variety of surgical areas, such as colorectal surgery, vascular surgery, thoracic surgery, and more recently radical cystectomy, and have led to a reduction in overall complications, decreased hospital stays, quicker resumption of bowel function, and an earlier return to the normal activities of daily living.

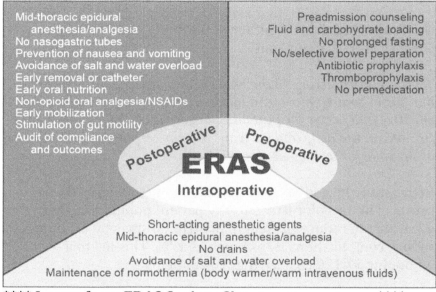

**** Image from ERAS Society Site: *http://erassociety.org*****

From this, the ERAS Society was formed in 2010 in Stockholm, Sweden as an offshoot of work by the ERAS Study Group. It has since spread internationally, and reflects a growing movement away from original surgical doctrine, and may potentially change the ways in which we counsel our patients both before and after surgery, as well as how we manage them during procedures themselves.

From my own review of the literature on surgical nutrition, it quickly became evident that the primary focus of most studies was that of hospitalized patients who were ultimately divided into those who the ERAS Study Group deemed to be nourished and those they described as severely malnourished. While the findings of these studies are legitimate, this focus is primarily on those undergoing in-patient procedures to the exclusion of those having surgery on outpatient bases. As discussed earlier, the trend toward outpatient surgeries is growing rapidly and embodies a huge number of surgical patients on an annual basis. Because many of these patients are ultimately assumed to be "healthy", no labs are ever drawn to evaluate nutritional parameters, and no educational guidance is given either before or after surgery.

To simply assume that every patient undergoing surgery is healthy and that all patients will consume healthy diets after their surgeries is assuming a lot. As the American diet continues to worsen and consumers become more and more confused about healthy dietary choices, this assumption may ultimately prove to undermine our patients' potential for optimal healing.

I am proud to say that the Cleveland Clinic Foundation (CCF), my alma mater, has made big strides in the last decade in changing not only the types of food fed to patients but also to family members, doctors, and employees. In September of 2015, under the guidance of Clinic Chief Executive and heart surgeon, Dr. Toby Cosgrove, CCF removed McDonald's® from its food court. Dr. Cosgrove had reportedly been on this course for over a decade but was locked in a battle with the local franchisee under the terms of its lease. "*We want to demonstrate that we can walk the talk by being a healthier organization*," said the spokeswoman, Eileen Sheil, who added that removing McDonald's is part of a much broader wellness campaign at the hospital.

Recently, while traveling through Toronto, Canada, I came across more evidence that hospitals are changing, not only within the United States, but also abroad. The Scarborough Hospital (TSH) launched the program "ReFRESHing Our Menu", a year-long project to improve food being fed to hospital patients.

This project removed much of the outsourced frozen products, replacing them with fresher, healthier, and apparently more appetizing food for their in-patient population and using locally sourced ingredients as available. According to **Dr. Tom Chan**, Chief of Staff at TSH, "*These aren't examples of average hospital food. They're freshly prepared meals featuring local ingredients and culturally diverse choices.*" He adds, "*We all like to complain about the food that we receive on airlines, because we really have no choice—that's the food that's there. And this is what happened with hospitals. When you show up to the hospital, you're expecting lukewarm tea, Jell-O pudding or the gelatinous goo that we used to serve our patients in plastic containers. Nobody ever looked forward to a meal like that.*"

Since instituting this novel program, the hospital has seen food waste drop by nearly a quarter and patient satisfaction scores regarding food rise. "*Fresher food looks more appealing, and if it doesn't have to travel a long distance to reach people's plates, the aromas, texture and taste are all enhanced,*" says **Rhonda Seldman Carson**, Vice President of Interprofessional Practice and Chief Nursing Executive at TSH.

Dr. Chan is quick to point out, "*Nobody questions the cost of drugs or the cost of surgery: if that's what somebody needs to get better, that's what they get. Yet we nickel and dime the costs of foods so painfully and completely miss the potential for food to help people recover when they are sick.*"

I believe **Chef Joshna Mahara**, the good-food advocate who led the menu overhaul, sums it up perfectly when she adds, "*We had food to cure us and heal us before we had medication.*"

As medical professionals, we need to come full circle and better appreciate the power of healthy food and the impact it has on our patients, both before and after surgery, as well as the implications it has for the general population of people simply trying to avoid disease. Instead of waiting for our patients to develop complications, we need to check nutritional statuses before surgeries, and we need to do so proactively through protocols built into our surgical systems.

You, the consumer, then need to bear responsibility for accepting these recommendations and implementing them into your pre-surgical planning. Without full compliance, protocols will have little to no effect, and we, as doctors, will be simply wasting our time. By working together, we can create better outcomes and get you back on your feet faster and with far less downtime.

How We Will Change Medicine: The Nutrition Revolution

"It is far more important to know what person the disease has than what disease the person has."
- **Hippocrates** (philosopher)

The goal of this book is not only to underscore the importance of nutrition in the healing process, but also to provide a framework from which you can design a pre- and post-recovery plan. While these tools are important, they are far more powerful when utilized in combination with the guidance and support of your doctor. Together, you can tailor a plan geared toward a speedy recovery following your surgery.

While many physicians are beginning to grasp the importance of nutrition, the vast majority is stuck in the past, with outdated information and protocols that lean far more towards technology than the basics of what we eat. That is why we need to change the way physicians work with patients. Technology will continue to be a critical element to success, but it is not the only one.

To affect change, the medical system needs to place more value on the nutritional training of young physicians from Day One. It needs to start that now. We need to look at surgical success as the combination of the Right Doctor, the Right Procedure, and the Right Internal Environment.

To create this environment, we need to think of the body as an engine, and provide it with the means to function as efficiently as possible far before complications ever arise. We need to look at the body before surgery (not after) and ask what is missing, what can be fine-tuned, and what additional nutrients will help provide the keys to success. As physicians, we spend a far greater time honing our skills for identifying and treating complications than we do preventing them. This cycle needs to stop. To achieve success, we need to implement three basic principles: EDUCATION, EMPHASIS, and EASE.

EDUCATION

First, there must be **EDUCATION**. Our patients must bear responsibility for lifestyle choices that will negatively impact their health and consider these to be detriments and potential sources of surgical complications.

As physicians, we must also take the reins and guide our patients toward better decisions in an effort to maximize their healing. And we must do this together.

Knowledge is power. You can no longer plead ignorance when it comes to your choices, and you must ask physicians to do the same. You also must allow physicians to be candid and to trust that they will guide you in a direction that is truly in your best interest. You must do so even when this change is hard. Science clearly shows that lifestyle choices contribute to many of the top disease processes, yet many Americans continue down a road that is unhealthy simply because it is easier. That has to change. Without change, tiny tweaks a week or two before surgery, while potentially positive, will have far less effect than changes made before you actually require surgery. Education, combined with personal responsibility, will ultimately prove to be far more powerful than either alone.

EMPHASIS

The next principle is **EMPHASIS**. We need to underscore the importance and the overriding value of a healthy diet from Day One. Elective surgeries aside, many of us will never be given ample time to prepare for our next procedures, so time is of the essence. Proper lifestyle choices must be made now, and they must be made with intent.

Physicians can no longer afford to side-step the fact that proper nutrition plays a role in how bodies function.

For too long, we physicians accepted improper and unhealthy lifestyle choices in the name of political correctness. In our efforts to be nice, we accepted mediocrity as we adjusted our language to avoid offending our patients. In doing this, our efforts have achieved quite the opposite. Chronically elevated blood sugars (a well-known side-effect of the typical American diet) have been clinically shown to cause disease, not only in the long-run, but also in the short-term, and have been shown to be a factor in compromised wound-healing. We need to address what you, our patients, are eating and its shortcomings, or we will be spending far more dollars healing complications after surgery than we ever imagined. And that is not good medicine.

EASE

The final principle is that of **EASE**. We need to simplify and demystify healthy eating. Too many Americans are confused by the vast amounts of conflicting information they read on a healthy diet. This confusion often leads to a virtual "paralysis of analysis", where nothing gets accomplished, and no change whatsoever is made. Easy access to a growing wealth of information related to health and wellness has turned what should have been a good thing into a virtual Pandora's Box. Open the lid on the Internet, and you may just be surprised what comes out. The food we eat is a drug. Taken correctly, it can heal us. Taken incorrectly and in the wrong amounts, it can ultimately hurt us...or worse.

According to a 2013 Journal of the American Medical Association study ("The State of US Health, 1990-2010: Burden of Diseases, Injuries, and Risk Factors." JAMA. 2013;310(6):591-606. doi:10.1001), the food we eat ranks as the single most important factor affecting premature death and disease.

According to several reports, only about a quarter of American medical schools offer the requisite 25 hours of training recommended (but not required) by the National Academy of Sciences. You will learn, however, that this sad state of affairs may soon be changing.

Although we have focused on many areas where the American medical system has potentially failed us, it is now time to look at a few areas where it is improving. In 2007, Harvard Medical School (HMS) and The Culinary Institute of America® (CIA) launched a collaborative effort entitled "*Healthy Kitchens, Healthy Lives: A Leadership Conference Bridging Nutrition Science, Health Care, and the Culinary Arts*".

This collaboration is aimed at educating healthcare professionals in the art of healthy eating through a series of seminars led by Harvard scientists and hands-on cooking workshops directly led by CIA chef-instructors.
It also aims to introduce participants to the latest scientific findings regarding diet and nutrition, combined with practical and healthy cooking skills, ideas, and inspiration.

While the goal is to educate healthcare providers, the real long-term strategy is to provide an educated medical force that educates its patients and disseminates this information across an even broader platform. In addition, the intent is to help develop physicians and other healthcare providers as models and leaders in this area to effect positive and long-term change.

"What if physicians and other medical professionals had the necessary skills to model healthy eating behaviors themselves? Wouldn't this impact their instructions and advice to their patients? Healthy Kitchens, Healthy Lives is intended to attract, inform, and inspire this and the next generation of medical professionals and food industry leaders to serve as role models for change when it comes to healthy eating."
 - **David M. Eisenberg, Bernard Osher**
Associate Professor/Harvard Medical School

In addition to providing broad information related to healthy foods, the conference goals hone in on a few "state-of-the-science" targeted areas, such as:

- Advice for diabetic patients about healthy carbohydrate choices
- Differentiating between "good" and "bad" fats
- Deconstruction of popular fad diets
- Mindfulness and exercise for weight management and healthy lifestyles
- Relationship between diet and cancer risks

Since its inception, the program has rapidly gained popularity and continues to be an event that sells out yearly.

"Our objective is to give physicians and other healthcare professionals the culinary tools to translate the best of nutrition science into flavorful, well-prepared meals, in the hope that they will be inspired to pass this new understanding on to their patients."
- **Dr. Tim Ryan**, President
The Culinary Institute of America

For real change to occur, it needs to be instituted much earlier in the training of our young physicians. A 2009 article published in the journal *Academic Medicine* found that "...only 25% of medical schools have a stand-alone nutrition course" (http://www.ncbi.nlm.nih.gov/pubmed/20736683), and concluded, *"The amount of nutrition education that medical students receive continues to be inadequate."*

In another article referring to the groundbreaking program at Tulane, a medical student was quoted as saying, "We basically learn to take care of patients when things go wrong, which is sad. I think that we need to learn how to be able to make nutritious meals and to discuss diet in an educated manner."

This student was speaking from experience, having come from a training program which was one of the first in the nation to look into the relationship between nutritional education of our young medical students and the ability to pass along this potentially life-changing information to their eventual patients.

In 2012, Tulane School of Medicine stepped forward and launched the nation's first culinary medicine program. Flash-forward to today, and the Goldring Center for Culinary Medicine, under the guidance of director Dr. Timothy Harlan, a chef-turned-internist, provides medical students with critical nutritional education through elective courses at the Center in addition to an exchange program with Johnson & Wales culinary school.

Since its launch, at least two other medical schools have licensed the Center's curriculum and are gearing up to introduce similar programs within the year.

The Tulane experience has stimulated the launch of a small, grant-funded pilot program at the University of Chicago, although at this time the program is off-campus and is not being offered for curriculum credit. This four-week pilot program begins its introduction with a one-hour overview on diet-related disease and how to treat it with food. From here, the students actually begin their hands-on training and begin to cook.

Another collaboration worth noting is that between the University of Ohio School of Medicine and Local Matters. Since 2011, this program has been teaching culinary/nutrition courses to medical students at the School of Medicine and is one of a small handful of known collaborations with the goal of educating our doctors on the importance of good nutrition and the science of it.

Medical students are not the only ones feeling the absence of proper nutrition in the American medical system. Board-certified cardiologist Dr. Stephen Devries left his cardiology practice a few years ago to launch the Gaples Institute, an effort aimed at expanding the nutrition training within medicine. He is reportedly expanding his efforts to launch an online course this summer that is geared towards nutritional training for doctors.

"I did a four-year, extra-intensive training program in cardiology and didn't receive one minute of training in nutrition. That's gotta stop".
- Stephen Devries, MD
Founder of the Gaples Institute

At a recent educational summit, Devries and other medical leaders met to discuss the importance of nutritional training and the steps necessary to integrate it into the training of our young physicians.

Another attendee, Dr. David Eisenberg, summed up it up perfectly : *"I don't think we could have predicted that health care professionals would need to know so much more about nutrition. Nor did we expect that we'd need to know more about movement and exercise or being mindful in the way we live our lives or eat or how to change behaviors."*
- Dr. David Eisenberg
Associate Professor of Nutrition Harvard, T.H. Chan School of Public Health
Executive Vice President, Health Research and Education, Samueli Institute

Change is achievable, but only if we work together. The American medical system needs to strip itself of antiquated beliefs and an overriding embrace of technology alone and accept the fact that some of the most basic building blocks for success often lie in the simplest things, such as food.

Consumers need to proactively educate themselves and bear responsibility for their actions. They need to press us, as physicians, to do the same. In the end, the journey toward optimal healing and surgical success may be decided by the simple step we take today toward changing what we eat. That, for all of us, is good medicine.

I hope that this information was helpful and that it literally changes your life. I look forward to hearing stories of your success and encourage you to contact me directly at drbuford@beautybybuford.com.

Be educated, be proactive, and (most of all) I wish that you be well. I leave you with the sage words of a fellow surgeon:

"Better is possible. It does not take genius. It takes diligence. It takes moral clarity. It takes ingenuity. And above all, it takes a willingness to try."
 - Atul Gawande, MD
Surgeon, Author
excerpt from Better: A Surgeon's Notes on Performance

How You Can Learn More

RESOURCES

My Favorite BLOGS

- Mark's Daily Apple
- MindBodyGreen
- Weighty Matters
- *The Atlantic* (articles by Dr. James Hamblin)
- The Kitchen
- Sprouted Kitchen
- 100 Days of Real Food
- Food Politics
- *Huffington Post*: Healthy Living
- Fit Men Cook

My Favorite Experts

With a wide array of apparent experts across the web, how do you know who to trust? I've listed my favorite top experts across the field of health and wellness and encourage you to check out their respective blogs, books, etc. If you know someone else who you feel is also a great resource, feel free to contact me directly with his or her name.

- Deepak Chopra
- Mark Sisson
- Gary Taubes
- Tim Ferriss
- Sanjay Gupta, MD
- Marion Nestle, PhD, MPH
- Michael Pollan
- Mark Hyman
- David Katz, MD, MPH
- Tony Robbins
- Joe Cross

- Joel Fuhrman, MD
- Yoni Freedhoff, MD
- Mark Sisson
- Frank Lipman, MD
- James Hamblin, MD
- Mike Roizen, MD

Expanded Micronutrient Analysis

The following is a more elaborate list of micronutrients, which can potentially optimize healing as well as improve your quality of life during the early weeks following your surgery. As stated previously, this list is significantly more comprehensive than the previous recommendations, so I suggest sticking with the basic list and adding on. Remember, bigger and more complicated is not always better. Start slow, and go from there.

Fat-soluble vitamins include the following:

☐ **Pro-Vitamin/Vitamin A**
- o Sources:
  - Spinach, broccoli, milk, eggs, liver, and fish
- o Functions:
  - Plays an essential role in vision, reproduction, cellular growth, and healthy immune function
- o Warnings:
  - Because these vitamins are stored in fat, high doses may ultimately lead to toxic levels and cause brain damage, etc.

- Low magnesium levels may hamper proper absorption.
  - o Recommended adult average daily dose range: 5,000 - 10,000 IUs

- ☐ **Vitamin D3**
  - o Sources:
    - Fatty fish, eggs, organ meats, milk, and sunlight
  - o Functions:
    - Thought to be more of a pro-hormone than an actual vitamin
    - Critical for maintaining proper blood levels of calcium by increasing calcium absorption from food and limiting calcium loss through urine
    - Important for maintaining healthy bones and teeth
    - May play a role in weight loss
    - Deficiencies can impact the optimal function of:
      - ☐ Immune system
      - ☐ Skin
      - ☐ Heart
      - ☐ Muscles
      - ☐ Brain

- o Warnings:
    - Because this vitamin is stored in body-fat tissue, high doses (around 50,000 IUs per day for a few months) can ultimately lead to toxic stored levels of Vitamin D and thereby cause excessive levels of calcium to circulate in the blood (hypercalcemia), which can lead to poor appetite, nausea, vomiting, and ultimately to soft-tissue calcium accumulation potentially in the arteries, kidneys, and other soft tissues.

- o Recommended adult average daily dose range: 1,000 - 2,000 IUs

- **Vitamin E (Alpha/Beta/Gamma-Tocopherol)**
    - o Sources:
        - Nuts and seeds, avocado, vegetables and vegetable oils, whole grains, organ meats, and eggs
    - o Functions:
        - Protection of cell membranes and other fat-soluble constituents of the body (e.g., LDL cholesterol)
        - May help reduce the risk of heart attacks
        - May play a role in the body's ability to process glucose, so may be helpful in prevention/treatment of diabetes
        - May directly affect inflammation, blood-cell regulation, connective tissue growth, and the genetic control of cellular division

- o Warnings:
    - Low chance of toxicity levels; however, due to the fact that these vitamins are stored in fat, high doses may possibly lead to toxic levels and symptoms such as nausea; diarrhea; stomach cramps; headache; blurred vision; rash; fatigue; weakness; and may cause hypervitaminosis E, which may increase bleeding and bruising problems and potentially lead to a Vitamin K deficiency.
- o Recommended adult average daily dose range: Controversial but safely 30 IUs (if alpha alone) - 400 IUs (if mixed carotenoids)
- ☐ **Vitamin K**
    - o Sources:
        - Leafy greens, nattō (fermented soy extract used in K2 supplement sourcing), synthesized by good bacteria in the GI tract
    - o Functions:
        - Comes in three forms: K1, K2 (recommended form), and K3
        - See previously in book for more details.
    - o Warnings:
        - ☐ Use with caution, and notify your healthcare practitioner if you are taking blood-thinning medications, such as COUMADIN®.
- o Recommended adult average daily dose range: 70-100 mcg (Vitamin K2)

Water-soluble vitamins include the following:

☐ **Vitamin B1 (Thiamine)**
- o Sources:
  - Whole grains, meat, nuts, yeast products, and legumes
- o Functions:
  - Required for the breakdown of carbohydrates, fats, and proteins
  - Essential component in the production of ATP (adenosine tri-phosphate) for energy
  - Critical to the proper functioning of nerve cells

- o Recommended adult average daily dose range: 1.1 to 8 mg, depending on gender, exercise levels, stress levels, and overall health

☐ **Vitamin B2 (Riboflavin)**
- o Sources:
  - Leafy-green vegetables, fish, eggs, dairy, meat and organ meats, nuts, and whole grains
- o Functions:
  - Important for the processing of amino acids and fats
  - Important for the activation of Vitamins B6/B9
  - Important component in the conversion of carbohydrates to ATP for energy
  - May act as an antioxidant under certain conditions
  - Warnings:

- Low toxicity levels
- Higher intake levels may harmlessly turn urine a brighter yellow color.
  - o Recommended adult average daily dose range: 1.67 to 4 mg

- **Vitamin B3 (Niacin)**
  - o Sources:
    - Poultry, meats, nuts, whole grains, fish, and dairy products
  - o Functions:
    - Required for cellular respiration
    - Critical component in the release of energy from carbohydrates, fats, and proteins
    - Important for the support of proper circulation, healthy skin, optimal functioning of the nervous system, and normal secretion of bile/stomach acids
    - May be effective in the treatment of schizophrenia and other mental illnesses
    - May enhance memory
  - o Warnings:
    - May cause skin flushing
    - Be careful using high doses for cholesterol-lowering and good HDL-increasing therapy. May increase the potential for liver damage
  - o Recommended adult average daily dose: 20 mg

- **Vitamin B5 (Pantothenic Acid)**
  - o Sources:

- Peas, beans, whole grains, meats, poultry, and fruits
- o Functions:
    - Plays an important role in the metabolism of and release of energy from sugar and fats
    - Important factor in the production of fats
    - Plays a role in modifying the shape of proteins
- o Warnings:
    - Low-level toxicity
- o Recommended adult average daily dose range: 20 mg

☐ Vitamin B6 (Pyridoxamine)

- o Sources:
    - Bananas, potatoes, meats and organ meats, fish, poultry, legumes, nuts and leafy-green vegetables
- o Functions:
    - Important component in the synthesis of antibodies by the immune system
    - Helps to maintain nervous system function
    - Aids in the formation of red blood cells
    - Critical component in chemical reactions necessary for digestion of proteins; the higher your protein intake, the more you require Vitamin B6.

o Warnings:

  ▪ Low level of toxicity or side effects if taken at recommended daily amounts. However, if higher daily amounts are taken, it may cause neurological disorders, lowered blood pressure, headaches, a rash, stomach discomfort, and sun sensitivity

o Recommended adult average daily dose range: 2 mg. to 10 mg.

☐ **Vitamin B9 (Folic Acid)**

o Sources:

o Eggs; dairy; asparagus; orange juice; dark, leafy-green vegetables; beans; brown bread; and tea

o Functions:

  ▪ Folate is naturally occurring in food; folic acid is the synthetic form.

  ▪ Important in the metabolism of amino acids and the production of proteins, nucleic acids, and blood cells

  ▪ Although folic acid has been shown to reduce homocysteine levels, its ability to reduce heart disease has been called into question in recent studies.

o Warnings:

  ▪ In normal doses, folate is very safe, but if given in mega-doses (usually above 15,000 mcg), you may experience stomach problems, sleep disturbance, skin reactions, and seizures.

- While it has been suggested to be preventative of various cancers, recent studies have suggested that it may actually increase progression of these cancers when they are already present. If you have a history of colon cancer or polyps, you may want to lower your intake of folic acid, since it could potentiate the growth of cancer by reducing the effectiveness of your body's own cancer-fighting "natural killer cells".

  o Recommended adult average daily dose:
    - 400 mcg/day
    - Should be taken on an empty stomach, since food may delay or reduce overall absorption
    - Higher doses may mask an underlying B12 deficiency.

- **Vitamin B12 (Cyanocobalamin or Superior Form, Methyl-Cobalamin)**
  o Sources:
    - Dairy products, eggs, fish, meats, and fermented foods
  o Functions:
    - Critical for nervous system function and replication of DNA
    - The active methyl component is utilized in the production of SAMe, which may be effective in the treatment of osteoarthritis as well as various mental disorders like depression.
    - Participates with folic acid to reduce homocysteine levels

- o Warnings:
  - If you have Leber's hereditary optic neuropathy (affecting your eyes), caution should be taken when consuming supplemental Vitamin B12. Avoid taking supplemental forms if allergic to cobalt or cobalamin.
- o Recommended adult average daily dose range: 50 to 100 mcg
  - Sublingual (dissolved underneath the tongue) methyl-cobalamin is most efficient for increased absorption, especially as you age and lose intrinsic factor production, and therefore have lowered GI absorption. Sublingual B12 can also help to positively support mental and physical relaxation and sleep quality.

☐ **Vitamin H (Biotin)**
- o Sources:
  - Dairy products, meat and poultry, oats and grains, soybeans and legumes, mushrooms, and nuts
- o Functions:
  - Actually considered to be a member of the Vitamin B family
  - Actively involved in energy production, as well as synthesis of fatty acids
  - Supports optimal nervous system function
- o Warnings:
  - A low level of toxicity and side effects
- o Recommended adult average daily dose: 300 mcg

□ **Vitamin C**

o Sources:

- Berries, fruits (especially citrus), red peppers, tomatoes, broccoli, spinach, and sprouts
- Camu camu berries are an excellent source!

o Functions:

- Potent antioxidant
- Protects LDL cholesterol (bad cholesterol) from oxidative damage
- Key component in collagen production
- Critical for optimal wound healing
- Aids in the formation of liver bile

o Warnings:

- High doses may cause gastrointestinal distress and diarrhea. Test for maximum dosage tolerability by implementing the Bowel Tolerance Test.

o Recommended adult average daily dose range: 60 mg (Daily value) to 2,000 mg+ (For some chronic illnesses, it can slow the progression of hardening of the arteries; for acute illnesses, like colds, sore throats, etc.)

MINERALS

☐ **Calcium**

o Sources:
- Dairy products, fish with bones, whole grains, seeds and nuts, green vegetables, and beans

o Functions:
- Aids in bone formation
- Required for proper blood clotting, signal transmission in nerve cells, and muscle contraction
- May play a role in lowering blood pressure

o Warnings:
- Calcium taken in excessive amounts can potentially cause soft tissue and vascular calcification, renal insufficiency, hypercalcemia, and kidney stones. To minimize these, balance appropriately your intake of calcium with appropriate amounts of magnesium, D3, K2, boron, etc.

o Recommended adult average daily dose range: 800 to 1,200 mg (depending on dietary intake, age, gender, bone health, etc.)

☐ **Chlorine**

o What:
- Mineral (present in the body as the chloride ion)

- o Sources:
  - Table salt, tap/bottled water, celery, tomatoes, seafood, pickled foods, and salted foods
- o Functions:
  - Essential to life
  - Responsible in part for the maintenance of membrane potential in nerves, nutrient absorption, and transport
  - Helps maintain proper balance of blood volume and pressure
- o Warnings:
  - Excessive amounts of chlorine in (sodium) chloride form may increase or exacerbate blood pressure in certain individuals.
- o Recommended adult average daily dose range: 1,800 to 2,300 mg

- ☐ **Chromium**
  - o Sources:
  - o Fermented foods, whole grains, dairy products, meats, grapes and raisins, beets, and black pepper

o Functions:

- Essential in production of glucose tolerance factor (GTF)
  - GTF is responsible for potentiating the effect of insulin and may actually help to lower blood-sugar levels, although results are inconclusive at this point.
  - It also may improve glucose transport into fat cells and muscle cells of the heart (cardiomyocytes).
- Active component in the synthesis of fatty acids and cholesterol

o Warnings:

- The polynicotinate form (as opposed to the picolinate form) in <u>some</u> studies may be safer and more absorbable.
- If diabetic and using medications to control blood sugars, consult with your healthcare practitioner before adding this supplement to your daily regimen.

o Recommended adult average daily dose range: 90 to 120 mcg

☐ **Copper**

o Sources:

- Seafood, whole grains and nuts, meats and organ meats, legumes and green vegetables, and molasses

- Functions:
  - Necessary for proper absorption and utilization of iron
  - Critical component in a number of varied chemical reactions throughout your body
- Warnings:
  - Some individuals are sensitive to even small amounts of supplemental copper intake, with short-term symptoms of nausea, vomiting, and diarrhea. However, copper toxicity is rare. For general health support and proper absorption, consume in an approximate nutrient balance of 1:15 with zinc. Therefore, if taking 1 mg of copper, also consume approximately 15 mg of zinc.
- Recommended adult average daily dose range: 750 mcg. to 2 mg.

□ **Magnesium**
- Sources:
  -
  - green vegetables, nuts and beans, and fruits
- Functions:
  - Necessary for the optimal formation of protein, bone, and fatty acids
  - Key component in cellular growth
  - Functions in the activation of B vitamins
  - Participates in the process of muscle relaxation, clotting of your blood, and formation of ATP for energy
  - May potentially lower blood pressure

o Warnings:
  - Magnesium blood toxicity (hypermagnesemia) is very rare and usually only occurs in certain chronically ill patients. (In fact, the latest nutritional information on magnesium is that most individuals are actually very <u>deficient</u> in this crucial mineral and could potentially increase their overall health and well-being by adding a magnesium supplement and/or increasing magnesium-rich foods in their diets.)

o Recommended adult average daily dose range: The new recommendation is closer to a 1:1 ratio with high-quality calcium or approximately 800 to 1,000 mg. (The old recommendation was closer to a 1:2 ratio with calcium or approximately 400 mg.)

☐ **Manganese**

o Sources:
  - Seeds and nuts, whole grains, green leafy vegetables, berries and fruit, eggs, avocado, tea, and seaweed

o Functions:
  - Required in small amounts for the manufacture of enzymes necessary in the metabolism of proteins and fat
  - Supports optimal immune system function, as well as blood-sugar balance
  - Participates in the production of cellular energy, reproduction, and bone growth
  - Works with Vitamin K to support normal blood clotting

- Warnings:
  - Low risk of toxicity, unless patient has long-term liver disease, iron-deficiency or anemia – these patients should have their dosages monitored closely
- Recommended adult average daily dose range: Adequate intake (AI) levels are 1.8 to 2.6 mg, depending on gender.

□ **Molybdenum**
- Sources:
  - Legumes; dark, leafy-green vegetables; whole grains; dairy products; and organ meats
- Functions:
  - Required for the activity of some enzymes involved in catabolism (including the breakdown of purines/sulfur amino acids)
- Warnings:
  - Low level of toxicity, unless exposed to a large amount of molybdenum in dust and fumes, primarily in mining and metalworking
- Recommended adult average daily dose: 75 mcg [Daily Value]

□ **Phosphorus**
- Sources:
- Fermented foods, meats and poultry, whole grains and seeds, dairy and eggs, mushrooms, and vegetables
  - Functions:
    - Usually found in nature combined with oxygen as "phosphate"

- Most phosphate in the body found in your bones
- Integral part of cell membranes (phospholipids) and lipoprotein molecules
- Trace amounts participate in biochemical reactions throughout your body.
  o Warnings:
    - Low level of toxicity
  o Recommended adult average daily dose range: 1,000 mg. (1 gram) [Daily Value]

☐ **Potassium**
  o What:
    - Macromineral
  o Sources:
    - Unprocessed meats; fish; milk; fruits and vegetables, such as leafy greens, bananas, berries, oranges, lemons, avocados, and tomatoes
    - Also found in fruit from vines and citrus
    - Highly refined food items such as oils, sugar, and fats lack potassium.
  o Functions:
    - Found in all cells of the body; levels controlled by kidneys
    - Essential mineral/electrolyte; helps regulate blood pressure and may reduce risk for cardiovascular disease
    - Plays an important role in electrolyte regulation, nerve function, muscle control

- Works with sodium to maintain blood pressure by increasing sodium excretion from the body
- Regulates water and mineral balance throughout the body

o Warnings:

- Excessive potassium intake rarely occurs within healthy individuals with properly functioning kidneys. Excess potassium in the body (hyperkalaemia) may occur in patients with renal disease (compromised kidney function), especially if given too much potassium chloride salt supplementation.
- Cardiovascular and neuromuscular abnormalities can occur with excessive body potassium levels.
- The safest and most natural way to obtain adequate levels of potassium is by consuming the whole foods mentioned above.

o Recommended adult average daily dose range:

- Most Americans do NOT get enough potassium in their diets.
- The adequate intake (AI) daily level range established for adults 18 years and older is 4,700 to 5,100 mg.

HERBS

☐ **Curcumin**

- o Sources:
    - Found in low levels in the herb turmeric. Because of these low levels, it is best to supplement with curcumin directly instead of turmeric.
- o Functions:
    - May be combined with black pepper/piperine to increase bioavailability (inhibitor of glucuronidation); can also increase bioavailability by creating nanoparticles, liposomes, micelles, and phospholipid complexes (advantages: longer circulation, increased cellular permeability, induced resistance to metabolic processes)
    - Bromelain increases the anti-inflammatory effect, so it is often combined with curcumin for increased effectiveness.
- o Warnings:
    - May increase the anti-platelet effect of various medications; check with your surgeon before taking this before or immediately following surgery.
    - May increase stomach acid. Clear with your primary physician if you have a history of reflux, stomach ulcers, or other intestinal issues.
    - Recommended adult average daily dose range: 500 mg, two times per day

- **Gotu Kola**
  - o What:
    - Herb
  - o Sources:
    - Capsules, loose herb powder
  - o Functions:
    - Wound healing/connective tissue production
  - o Daily dosage: Standardized 30 - 90 mg

- **Chamomile**
  - o What:
    - Herb
  - o Sources:
    - Flower buds, tea
  - o Functions:
    - Has calming effect, internally and topically
    - Immune booster
  - o Dosage: In capsule form, 400 to 1600 mg per day
    - Can consume in tea form and/or use soaked chamomile teabags topically for soothing/healing properties

- **Calendula (Marigolds)**
  - o What:
    - Herb
  - o Source:
    - Topical cream

- Functions:
  - Promotes wound-healing
  - Soothes topically
- Dosage:
  - Limited evidence is available, but applying a prepared, topical calendula cream throughout the day for soothing and healing purposes is acceptable.

- **Quercetin**
  - What:
    - Flavonol antioxidant
  - Sources:
    - Buckwheat, onions, citrus fruits, berries
  - Functions:
    - Potent flavonoid
    - Reduces swelling and lymphedema
    - Blood vessel protection and support
    - Allergy reaction support
  - Dosage: 500 mg, two times per day

- **Ginger**
  - What:
    - A rhizome
  - Sources:
    - Capsules, tea, powder
  - Functions:
    - GI calming effect
    - Anti-inflammatory
    - May thin blood

o Dosage:

- Best to use fresh-cut pieces for optimal enzyme and antioxidant activity or drink as a tea
- 250 mg - 2 g of powder extract or in encapsulation

Chlorella

o What:

- Single-celled plant

o Sources:

- Capsules, dry powder, liquid

o Functions:

- Speeds up cell growth and wound-repair
- Blood purifier

o Daily dosage: 2 grams total in either capsule, powder, or liquid form

Garlic

o What:

- Herb

o Sources:

- Fresh, capsules, powder, oil, extracts

o Functions:

- Antioxidant
- Reduces infection
- Liver detoxification
- May increase bleeding

o Dosage: 2 to 5 g fresh, raw garlic; 0.4 to 1.2 g dried garlic powder; 2 to 5 mg garlic oil; 300 to 1,000 mg garlic extract

- **Ginkgo Biloba**
  - o What:
    - Herb
  - o Sources:
    - Capsules
  - o Functions:
    - Antioxidant
    - Boosts circulation
  - o Daily dosage: 50 - 160 mg standardized extract

- **Bromelain**
  - o What:
    - Dietary enzyme derived from pineapple
  - o Sources:
    - Supplemental form or consumed directly in pineapple
  - o Functions:
    - Reduces swelling and inflammation
  - o Dosage: 90 mg, three times per day

- **Milk Thistle**
  - o What:
    - Herb
  - o Functions:
    - Antioxydant
    - Increases glutathione
    - Liver support
  - o Dosage: 50 to 300 mg standardized, two to three times per day, depending on your health, dietary

habits and lifestyle, and/or need to cleanse the liver

- **Echinacea**
  - o What:
    - Herb
  - o Sources:
    - Capsules, teas
  - o Functions:
    - Boosts immune system
    - Increases NK cell production and activity
  - o Daily dosage: 100 to 1,500 mg standardized extract in capsule or tea form

- **Grape Seed Extract**
  - o What:
    - Herb
  - o Sources:
    - Capsules, powders
  - o Functions:
    - Supports microcirculation
    - Improves capillary resistance
    - Reduces swelling
  - o Daily dosage: 100 to 150 mg standardized extract

- **Holy Basil(Tulsi)**
  - o What:
    - Herb/adaptogen
  - o Functions:
    - Improves response to stress
    - Potentially modulates cortisol

- Dosage: 100 - 300 mg standardized per day
  - Take when dealing with extra emotional stress and anxiety
- **Ashwaganda**
  - What:
    - Herb/adaptogen
  - Functions:
    - Improves response to stress
    - Potentially modulates cortisol
    - Potential neuron (brain cell) protector
  - Dosage: 50 to 500 mg, depending on goal

- **Green Tea (Epigallocatechin Gallate or EGCG)**
  - What:
    - Herb
  - Sources:
    - Powder, capsules, tea
  - Functions:
    - Potent catechins/EGCG phytochemical content with the following potential roles/functions:
    - Antioxidant
    - Anti-carcinogenic
    - Anti-inflammatory
    - Blood-sugar stabilizing
    - Thermogenic (fat-burning)
    - Increases focus and calmness via thiamine content

- Dosage: Daily intake of 3 to 5 cups per day (1,200 mL) of green tea provides at least 250 mg per day of catechins. (However, green tea extract should not be taken on an empty stomach, due to the potential for hepatotoxicity from excessive levels of epigallocatechin gallate [EGCG].)
    - Cardiovascular effect: 400 to 716 mg per day of catechins has been used in trials in divided dosages.
    - Diabetes: Dosages of EGCG range from 84 to 386 mg per day in trials evaluating glucose homeostasis.
    - Dosage ranges used in trials include 270 to 800 mg per day of EGCG or 125 to 625 mg per day of catechins.

☐ **Cayenne (Capsicum)**
- What:
    - Spice/pepper
- Functions:
    - May help improve blood-sugar control
    - May support blood vessel circulation
    - May support, in conjunction with other nutrients, a reduction in muscle and joint pain
- Dosage: Standardized 450 mg capsules, one to three times per day, preferably with food; or use in powder/spice form, and add to meals

☐ **Cloves**
- What:
    - Herb

o Sources:

- Powder, capsules

o Functions:

- Antibiotic function
- Natural COX-2 inhibitor (may increase bleeding or potentiate other substances that do)

o Dosage: Very strong; need only a 'pinch' or 1 to 2 capsules of even non-standardized extracts in tea, smoothies, taken with a glass of water, etc. to potentially achieve antioxidant/COX-2 inhibition effect

☐ **Coriander**

o What:

- Herb

o Sources:

- Powder, capsules

o Functions:

o Antioxidant

o Anti-anxiety effects

o Dosage: Use as desired in cooking.

☐ **Sage**

o What:

- Herb

o Sources:

- Powder, in combination anti-inflammatory formulas

o Functions:

- May reduce blood sugar
- May improve alertness

- Anti-inflammatory
- Antioxidant
o Dosage: Dried sage leaf has been investigated in studies on memory at doses of 300 and 600 mg per day. Ethanolic extract at 333 mg per day has been studied in Alzheimer's disease.
  - Typical medicinal dosage in the loose-tea-leaf form averages out to 4 to 6 g per day.

OTHER SUPPLEMENTS

- **Omega-3 Fatty Acids:**
  - o What:
    - PUFA (poly-unsaturated fatty acid)
  - o Sources: Flaxseeds, chia seeds, walnuts, fatty fish, grass-fed beef, flax-seed fed chicken eggs
  - o Functions:
    - After consumption of plant-based ALA, it is then converted to bioactive forms DHA and EPA in the body.
    - Comprised of ALA, DHA, and EPA
    - ALA omega3 (alpha linolenic acid)
  - o Sources:
    - Vegetable oils, including those from flaxseed, walnuts, and spinach
    - Our bodies cannot make ALA, so we must get it from our diets. However, under the right conditions, our bodies can convert ALA to DHA and EPA. This becomes important in the case of strict vegans, who cannot get DHA or EPA from their diets.
    - The problem with this is that the specific types of foods that we eat may not enable us to effectively convert ALA to DHA/EPA. This issue is rather complex.
    - The easiest option is to simply eat foods high in DHA/EPA or consume supplements that actually contain them.

- **DHA omega-3** (docosahexaenoic acid)
  - o Sources:

- Marine oils, including those from cold-water, oily fish; calamari; krill; marine algae; and phytoplankton
- DHA is naturally found throughout the body but is most abundant in the brain, eyes, and heart.
- This critical fatty acid is essential for optimal function and development of cells in the brain, retina, heart, and other parts of the nervous system.
- As a critical structural component of the brain, DHA makes up approximately 30% of the structural fats in the gray matter of the brain and 97% of the overall omega-3s in the brain.
- DHA is also a major structural fat in the retina of the eye. As such, it plays an important role in both infant visual development and visual function throughout life.
- Finally, DHA is a key component of the heart (especially in the conducting tissue) and is important for heart health throughout life.

o Studies have shown that DHAs play active roles in the following:
- Infant mental development
- Optimal brain and nervous system development and function
- Infant visual function and development of vision
- Maintenance of normal triglyceride levels, heart rate, and blood pressure
- Possible role in health of the adult eye

- Possible role in some behavioral and mood disorders affecting both children and adults
- Possible reduction of the risk of cardiovascular disease (Research at this point is inconclusive.)

☐ **EPA omega-3** (eicosapentaenoic acid)

o Sources:

- Marine oils, including those from cold-water, oily fish; calamari; krill; marine algae; and phytoplankton
- DHA in fish oils may lower elevated triglyceride levels.

o In general, fish oils may help with the following:

- Lowering of triglycerides
- Reduction of stiffness and joint pain associated with rheumatoid arthritis; may also boost overall effectiveness of various anti-inflammatory drugs
- On their own, they have helped reduce symptoms associated with depression and bipolar disorder, in addition to boosting the effects of various anti-depressant medications.
- Given their ability to lower overall inflammation, they may prove helpful in the treatment of asthma.

- Some recent studies suggest that fish oil may reduce the symptoms of ADHD in children and improve overall mental and cognitive skills.
- Some recent studies suggest that fish oils may help protect against Alzheimer's disease and dementia, in addition to having a positive effect on the progression of memory loss associated with aging.

o Warnings:
- Fish oils are known to have an anti-platelet effect, so they may increase your risk for bleeding. Fish oils should be stopped at least two weeks prior to surgery and continued only with the guidance of your treating physician.
- Know the source of your omega-3 fatty acids. This pertains more to DHA and EPA, which are generally sourced from cold-water fish, which may contain high levels of mercury and other potential contaminants.

o Recommended dosages: The FDA has advised that adults may safely consume a total of three grams per day of combined EPA/DHA, with no more than two grams coming from dietary supplements.

- **L-Glutamine**
  - What:
    - Free-form amino acid or found naturally or added to protein powders as glutamine peptides
  - Sources:
    - Supplemental amino acid or in protein powders
  - Functions:
    - Intestinal lining support
    - Immunity support
    - Promotes building of muscle
  - Dosage: 1 - 5 g, depending on specific goal

- **Zinc**
  - What:
    - Essential trace mineral
  - Sources:
    - Animal protein, beans, pumpkin seeds
  - Functions:
    - Immune support, fatty acid metabolism, acute infection support, growth and repair of cells and various body tissue
  - Recommended adult average daily dose range: 10 to 18 mg, depending on age and gender
    - Short-term immune support therapeutic dosage: 20 to 50 mg

- **Bioflavonoids**
  - o What:
  - o Antioxidant/phytochemical
  - o Sources:
    - Citrus fruits, buckwheat
  - o Functions:
    - Helps protect the body from oxidation
    - Supports the integrity of blood vessels
    - Works synergistically with Vitamin C
  - o Recommended adult average daily dose range: 100 to 500 mg

- **CoQ10**
  - o What:
    - Vitamin-like nutrient naturally produced in the body
  - o Sources:
    - Supplemental form, either as ubiquinol or ubiquinone; also naturally occurring in smaller amounts, animal-based proteins
  - o Function:
    - Antioxidant
    - Boosts intra-cellular energy
  - o Dosage: 50 to 200 mg

☐ **Probiotic**

   o What:

- Beneficial bacteria (or body flora) that resides primarily in the (upper) small intestine and the (lower) large intestine or colon, as well as other areas of the body

   o Sources:

- Supplemental form; fermented food products, such as kombucha, kimchi, and yogurt

   o Functions:

- Helps to support bowel regularity
- Supports immune system
- Creates proper upper and lower gastrointestinal pH balance
- To produce certain nutrients, especially some B vitamins

   o Dosage: Usually 1 to 100 billion colonizing units per day, depending on goals and/or conditions

☐ **Cinnamon**

   o What:

- Spice

   o Sources:

- Powder, capsules, tea

   o Functions:

- Antibiotic function
- Antioxidant
- Blood-sugar stabilization

o Dosage: Standardized 500 to 1,000 mg capsules, one to six times per day, preferably with food; or use in tea and/or add to smoothies

Results of Our Online Nutritional Survey

"The physician should not treat the disease but the patient who is suffering from it." - **Maimonides** (philosopher)

To better understand the importance that you, the consumer, actually place on proper nutrition, we did a crazy thing. We actually asked you!

To gauge public opinion, we designed and distributed a nutritional survey across a broad mix of social media platforms, presenting various questions related to both the importance of surgical nutrition and the degree of responsibility that you, as the potential patient, accept versus the responsibility you think should be borne by your physician. While participation was limited to just over 200 respondents, the results were fairly consistent.

You sent a strong message that nutrition is important and that both you and your doctor play important roles in determining which foods you should eat before and after surgery. You also felt that the medical profession, as a whole, is not as responsive as it should be.

You were asked to respond to questions on a sliding scale (from 1-5) ranging from "strongly disagree" to "strongly agree". Your answers were very telling.

Q1: Have you ever had surgery? A majority of respondents previously had surgery, while the remaining minority had not. This suggests that the answers received came predominantly from a population that actually previously experienced not only a surgical procedure but also the process leading up to it and the healing period following it.

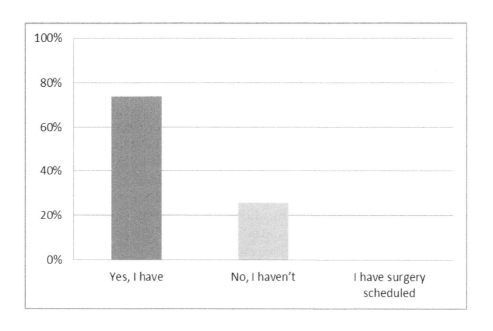

Answer	Response	
Yes, I have	148	74.00%
No, I haven't	52	26.00%
I have surgery scheduled	0	0.00%

Answered: 200 Skipped 1

Q2: Proper nutrition reduces complications after surgery.

The majority response was that proper nutrition DOES reduce complications after surgery. This being said, it only makes sense that you should be educated on what to eat (and what not to eat) before and after surgery to help improve your chances of optimal healing and reduce complications associated with your surgical procedure.

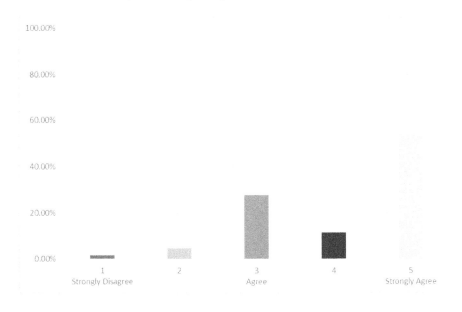

1	2	3	4	5
Strongly Disagree		Agree		Strongly Agree
3	9	53	22	104
1.57%	4.71%	27.75%	11.52%	54.45%

Answered: 191 Skipped: 10 Weighted Average: 4.13

Q3: Food affects the way you heal. The majority response was that food DOES affect the way you heal. Again, you felt that what you eat before and after surgery does make a difference and is an important factor in determining your post-surgical healing.

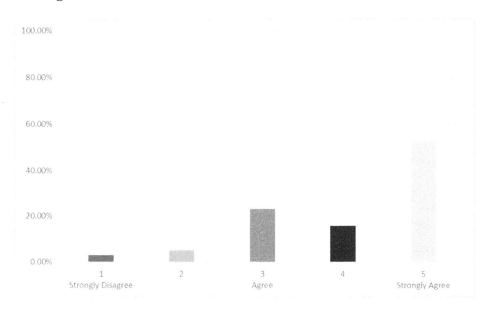

1	2	3	4	5
Strongly Disagree		Agree		Strongly Agree
6	10	44	30	101
3.14%	5.24%	23.04%	15.71%	52.88%

Answered: 191 Skipped: 10 Weighted Average: 4.10

Q4: Certain foods are more important for healing. Not surprisingly, you also felt that certain foods are more important for healing. This suggests that knowing what to eat may directly affect your healing.

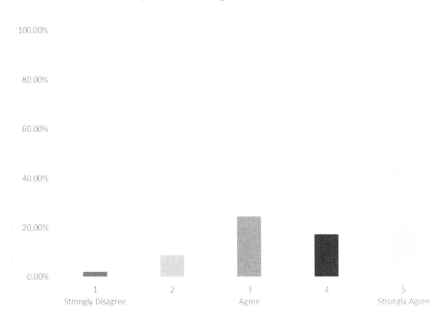

1	2	3	4	5
Strongly Disagree		Agree		Strongly Agree
4	17	47	33	89
2.11%	8.95%	24.74%	17.37%	46.84%

Answered: 190 Skipped: 11 Weighted Average: 3.98

Q5: Vitamins and other supplements are important for healing. You also felt that vitamins and other supplements are important for healing. This is a critical statement. Many consumers are overwhelmed with studies suggesting that supplementation is simply a waste of time. You felt otherwise. The real question is: If supplements really are important, which ones should you be taking, and what is the science behind their importance?

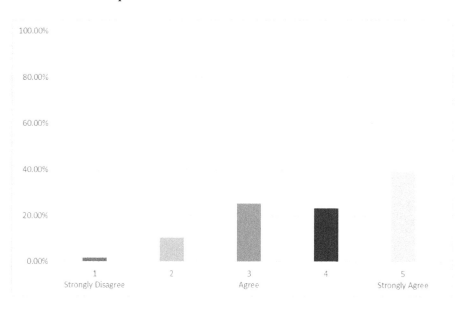

1	2	3	4	5
Strongly Disagree		Agree		Strongly Agree
3	20	48	44	75
1.58%	10.53%	25.26%	23.16%	39.47%

Answered: 190 Skipped: 11 Weighted Average: 3.88

Q6: Patients are responsible for educating themselves about proper nutrition before surgery. Here the results were mixed. While some of you thought that responsibility should be placed on the patient, others were not so sure. Feedback was more closely aligned in the middle for this question.

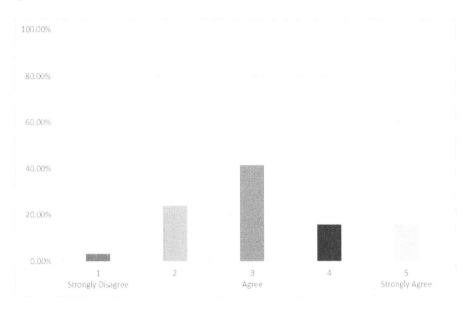

1	2	3	4	5
Strongly Disagree		Agree		Strongly Agree
6	43	75	28	29
3.31%	23.76%	41.44%	15.47%	16.02%

Answered: 181 Skipped: 20 Weighted Average

Q7: Doctors should be teaching patients about proper nutrition before surgery. You definitely responded differently here. A majority of study participants strongly agreed that this is the doctor's responsibility, with only a few suggesting that it is not. While you thought that patients should play a role, it appears that you felt the doctor's role should be even greater.

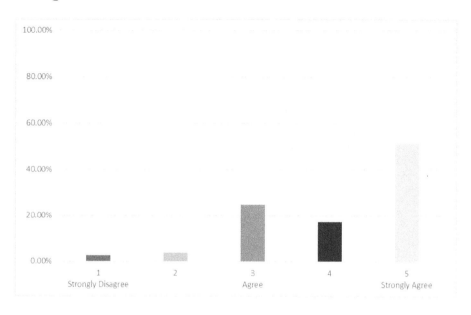

1	2	3	4	5
Strongly Disagree		Agree		Strongly Agree
5	7	45	31	93
2.76%	3.87%	24.86%	17.13%	51.38%

Answered: 181 Skipped: 20 Weighted Average: 4.10

Q8: Doctors are motivated to teach patients about proper nutrition before surgery. Most of you felt that doctors are NOT motivated to teach their patients about proper nutrition. That's a problem. This answer alone underscores the importance of a book such as this that not only helps educate you on the importance of surgical nutrition, but also provides you with a framework with which to design your surgical meal plan for the period leading up to and the period following your procedure.

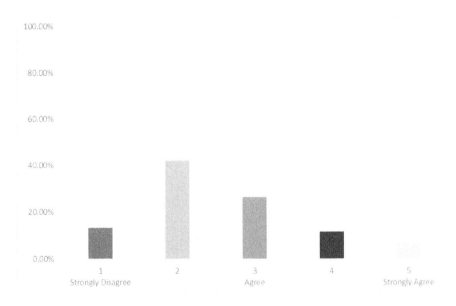

1	2	3	4	5
Strongly Disagree		Agree		Strongly Agree
24	76	48	21	12
13.26%	41.99%	26.52%	11.60%	6.63%

Answered: 181 Skipped: 20 Weighted Average: 2.56

Q9: Your doctor should look for nutritional deficiencies before surgery. A strong majority of you agreed that it is your doctor's responsibility to identify any nutritional deficiencies before surgery. I agree. Given the fact that many Americans either don't know what to eat on a normal basis or simply choose not to eat in a healthy manner; a problem arises when your body is placed under increased stress, such as the stress associated with surgery itself and the healing period that follows. If you are not optimized before surgery, then you enter a period of increased demand for optimal nutrition from a standpoint of depletion and potential malnutrition. The science clearly shows that this is a setup for failure from the start.

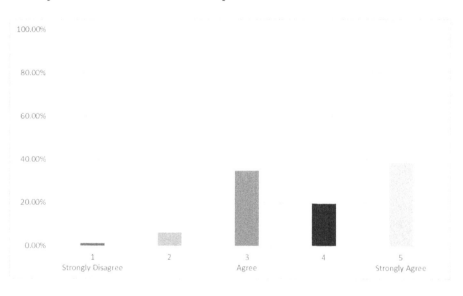

1	2	3	4	5
Strongly Disagree		Agree		Strongly Agree
19	71	56	21	13
10.56%	39.44%	31.11%	11.67%	7.22%

Answered: 179 Skipped: 22 Weighted Average: 3.88

Q10: The medical profession cares about proper nutrition for surgical patient. While slightly under half of you agreed with this statement, more than half did not. This is concerning. As physicians, we need to align ourselves with patients in a way in which they feel cared for and supported. If a majority of you feel that we simply don't care, there may be a disconnect in the care that we are providing for you.

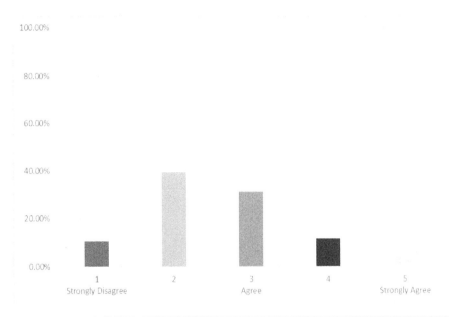

1 Strongly Disagree	2	3 Agree	4	5 Strongly Agree
19	71	56	21	13
10.56%	39.44%	31.11%	11.67%	7.22%

Answered: 180 Skipped: 21 Weighted Average: 2.66

Q11: Gender Women were significantly more represented than men, which may reflect a study bias. As a plastic surgeon, most of my patients are women. Therefore, for my patient population, this demographic detail is actually more appropriate. For a more accurate assessment, I would like to see increased input from men to see if they agree with these statements or if there is potentially a gender bias in the results.

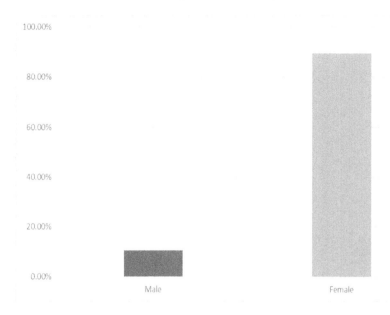

Answer	Response	
Male	19	10.61%
Female	160	89.39%

Answered: 179 Skipped: 22

Q12: Ethnicity a strong majority of respondents were Caucasian, which may also reflect a potential study bias. I spread this study across a broad range of popular social networks to reduce this potential bias; nonetheless, this may also reflect a potential flaw in the study. To address this, I plan to specifically target more ethnic respondents in the future.

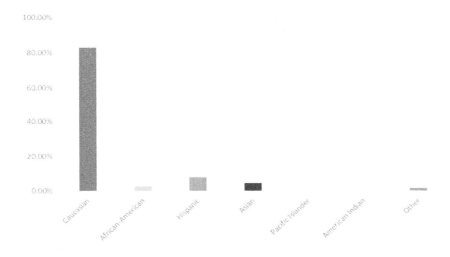

Answer	Response	
Caucasian	147	83.05%
African-American	5	2.82%
Hispanic	14	7.91%
Asian	8	4.52%
Pacific Islander	0	0.00%
American Indian	0	0.00%
Other	3	1.69%

Answered: 177 Skipped: 24

Q13: Age A majority of respondents were between the ages of 41 and 50, but there was a nice bell curve, which did include respondents as young as 1 to 18 years of age and as old as 70+. Again, future surveys will try to target a more age-specific range to see if there is an age-related bias tied to specific age groups.

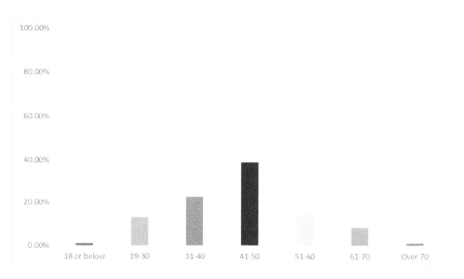

Answer	Response	
18 or below	2	1.12%
19-30	24	13.48%
31-40	40	22.47%
41-50	69	38.76%
51-60	26	14.61%
61-70	15	8.43%
Over 70	2	1.12%

Answered: 178 Skipped: 23

Q14: Education Over half of respondents had at least a college degree, with almost a quarter acknowledging a post-graduate degree. There were no participants identified as having no education at all.

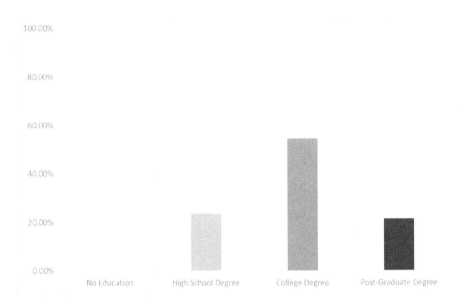

Answer	Response	
No Education	0	0.00%
High School Degree	42	23.73%
College Degree	97	54.80%
Post-Graduate Degree	38	21.47%

Answered: 177 Skipped: 24

Q15: Where do you live? A majority of participants lived in either the West Coast/Pacific Northwest or in the Midwest, with about half of the remaining people distributed across the East Coast and the South. Again, I would have liked a more even distribution, and this suggests the need for additional targeted surveying to identify a potential regional bias.

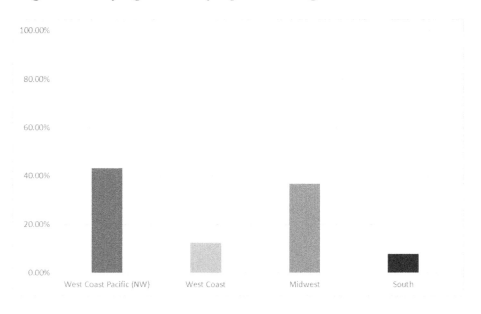

Answer	Response	
West Coast Pacific (NW)	77	43.26%
West Coast	22	12.36%
Midwest	65	36.52%
South	14	7.87%

Answered: 178 Skipped: 23

Q16: Annual income. Respondents were distributed across the salary range in a fairly even bell curve, with the median located in a broad range from a $50,000 to a $250,000 annual income, which suggests a more focused response from those in the middle to upper-middle income bracket.

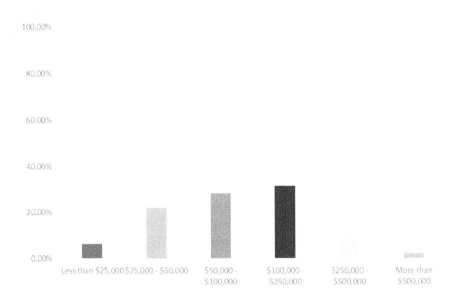

Answer	Response	
Less than $25,000	11	6.18%
$25,000 - $50,000	39	21.91%
$50,000 - $100,000	50	28.09%
$100,000 - $250,000	56	31.46%
$250,000 - $500,000	18	10.11%
More than $500,000	4	2.25%

Answered: 178 Skipped: 23

With your feedback, you sent a strong message. Although I am not surprised by the answers, I am disheartened, but also challenged. Part of me was hoping that I overestimated the concern that you, the public, have with the medical profession. Unfortunately, you proved my thesis correct. With this, the importance of this information is underscored and my efforts supported.

While on many levels we have an amazing medical system that provides amazing care, on others we are woefully lacking in what we provide to you, our patients. As the demand for technology increases, we have forgotten the basics that may, in the end, come back to haunt us. As physicians, we need to look at the whole patient, and not merely the diagnosis. We need to understand that the nutritional environment that our patients bring with them plays a huge role in how they heal, and that we simply cannot be so cavalier in our efforts at practicing medicine. A patient is a person and a whole being, not merely a diagnosis. Once we identify and embrace this change in thinking, we will be firmly set in a new direction that will truly benefit our patients and their long-term health. At the most fundamental level, that is practicing good medicine.

Made in United States
North Haven, CT
26 March 2023

34581026R00114